Understanding Epilepsy

Understanding Epilepsy

Second Edition

George Burden, OBE, BSc(Econ)

Secretary-General, International Bureau for Epilepsy,
1969-77, and Education Secretary to the British Epilepsy
Association, 1969-78

Peter H. Schurr, MA, MB, FRCS

Director, Neurosurgical Unit of Guy's, Maudsley and
King's College Hospitals, London

GRANADA
London Toronto Sydney New York

Granada Publishing Limited
Frogmore, St Albans, Herts AL2 2NF
and
3 Upper James Street, London W1R 4BP
Suite 405, 4th Floor, 866 United Nations Plaza, New York,
    NY 10017, USA
117 York Street, Sydney, NSW 2000, Australia
100 Skyway Avenue, Rexdale, Ontario M9W 3A6, Canada
PO Box 84165, Greenside, 2034 Johannesburg, South Africa
61 Beach Road, Auckland, New Zealand

First published by Crosby Lockwood Staples 1976
Second edition published by Granada Publishing 1980

ISBN 0 246 11353 7

Printed in Great Britain by
Richard Clay (The Chaucer Press) Ltd,
Bungay, Suffolk

Granada ®
Granada Publishing ®

Contents

Foreword to the First Edition

Desmond A. Pond, MA, MD, FRCP
Professor of Psychiatry, The London Hospital Medical College,
University of London.

Caring for people suffering from epilepsy often needs the combined efforts of different medical specialists and numerous other professionals, such as social workers and psychologists. Above all, the family of the sufferer very frequently needs specific advice and also the opportunity to share the worries and anxieties inevitably resulting from trying to deal with someone whose handicap is likely to be long term. The authors of this book have many years' experience in the care of people with epilepsy and they write out of their deep experience and wise reflection on the problems that they have faced and tried to solve. I have no doubt that their words will enable many sufferers and their families to achieve a happier and more successful adjustment.

Desmond A. Pond
April, 1975

Preface to the Second Edition

The first edition of this book aimed to tell the non-medical reader about the problems of those who suffer from epilepsy and how it may affect their social relationships. It was written primarily for those who need to know how to assess and react to these problems when they meet them as teachers, employers, family or friends. In the present edition the scope has been widened to include those who have found themselves to be suffering from epilepsy, whether as the result of a head injury, as a sequel to some other illness, or as a spontaneous occurrence for which there is no obvious cause, but the book's main purpose remains as before. It is not intended to be a guide to treatment, which must be in the hands of those who specialise in the subject. The authors hope that the book will foster a better understanding of how to respond to people who have this disability, and that it will encourage those who suffer from epilepsy to adjust themselves to the limitations it imposes. They hope also to show that even if fits cannot be completely suppressed or prevented in every case, adaptation to the situation can be achieved.

G. Burden
Peter H. Schurr, 1979

The authors are grateful to Dr M. V. Driver for the EEG records reproduced in this book and to Dr R. D. Hoare for the CT Scan, and patients and friends who have given them so much help.

CHAPTER ONE

The Problem

Epilepsy has been known throughout history. It observes no cultural, geographical or racial boundaries. Hundreds of thousands of men, women and children all over the world suffer from epilepsy, the occurrence of which is often unknown even to their friends. There are many people with epilepsy who hold responsible positions in society, and some have been among its leaders. Today we have the means of eliminating attacks altogether, or at least of reducing their frequency. Yet superstitions and old wives' tales persist, so much so that social attitudes towards the disorder are sometimes harder for the sufferer to bear than the condition itself.

Epilepsy occurs as a result of changes in the normal activity of certain brain cells. The extent of these changes, and their effect on the individual, varies from those which are so slight as to be undetectable without analysis of the electrical activity of the brain, to major seizures in which there are convulsions and loss of consciousness. All are degrees of the same phenomenon. The words 'fit', 'attack' or 'seizure' mean the same thing. They have no significance with regard to the severity of the event. Whether the patient loses consciousness or not, and whether he convulses or merely stares in the attack, is irrelevant. These are all epileptic fits.

Some people are more susceptible to attacks than others, but nobody is immune to the possibility of them. Anyone can have fits after a serious head injury, or as a result of changes in the blood chemistry; some may have them on account of brain tumours and a variety of other causes outlined in Chapter 4, but in the majority of cases no reason for the fits can be demonstrated apart from the existence of a greater susceptibility to fits than average. Medicines given for treatment of epilepsy are designed to decrease that susceptibility, hopefully restoring the situation to normal. The varieties of fit which can occur are considered, and treatment is referred to in Chapters 3 and 4, but this is not a textbook on epilepsy, of which there are many, and possibilities for further reading are given at the end of this book.

Society finds it difficult to accept any behaviour which appears to be outside voluntary control, or any apparently unprovoked impairment of consciousness. But because fits are so common it is essential that everyone should know more about them and how to react in the presence of an attack. If the public were better informed about the disorder, people with epilepsy and their relatives would be less anxious and more able to stand up to their difficulties; needless apprehension on the part of employers, teachers and others might also be allayed.

Generally speaking, a mother quickly learns how to look after a child who has epilepsy, but as he grows older and moves into the community he leaves that highly protected environment. It should be a normal part of teacher-training to know how to treat a pupil with a fit without creating anxiety in others and with assurance that the child can be protected from harm. It is important for a headmaster to know how to integrate someone with epilepsy into the normal curriculum, and what effect his presence will have (or not have) on both pupils and staff.

When epilepsy occurs at an age at which it is normal to be employed, it is necessary for many people (including employers, managers, personnel officers, foremen and colleagues) to understand the capabilities of the person who has fits, to realise that most attacks are very intermittent and that the sufferer is likely to be quite normal at other times. It is important not to penalise him as a result of excessive caution, but at the same time he must not be a source of danger to himself or others, nor must he throw an extra burden on those who work with him. Opportunities are too often closed unnecessarily, without careful consideration or assessment of the facts. Valuable services are thereby lost to the community and the sufferer is given a further and unjust burden to bear. There are about 300,000 people in the United Kingdom who have epileptic seizures and this large number cannot simply be discarded. This is particularly clear when one considers that two-thirds of them have their fits controlled by regular medication and rarely have an attack.

Personal relationships are often marred if it is known that someone has fits. This may simply be a matter of ignorance or prejudice, and it is the aim of this book to clear up such misunderstandings. However, special problems arise with marriage. Both partners need guidance and encouragement in the face of a problem which has to be shared, and which requires an understanding and sensitive approach, not only by those most immediately concerned, but also by newly acquired friends and relatives. Questions about the possibility of epilepsy occurring in children are bound to arise, and the misinformed are usually only too ready to spread unwarranted gloom and despondency (p. 83).

Our hope is that this book may clear up some misconceptions and promote a better understanding of the condition called epilepsy, which is not a word to be avoided or a disease to be shunned, but a natural event that unfortunately occurs too readily in some people. Lack of familiarity and apprehension have perpetuated an attitude of rejection from the time when people with epilepsy were endowed with supernatural powers (and there are plenty of examples of this belief in most religions), down to the present day.

When a rational and often highly intelligent person behaves in a manner that is clearly abnormal, it naturally gives rise to a sense of mystery and lack of comprehension. If his behaviour should at times appear violent, even if that violence is limited to purposeless movement, it is not surprising that it should cause fear, and a desire to be rid of the situation. We are unlikely to be able to change these attitudes overnight, but with greater understanding of the nature of epilepsy, society should acquire tolerance and acceptance of it.

If you are yourself liable to attacks, this book may help you to gain the confidence of other people, or to regain your own. If you can explain what special considerations may be necessary with regard to yourself, while at the same time demonstrating your capabilities and maintaining an enthusiasm for life, you will find most people prepared to listen and help. An epilepsy association probably exists in your own country and may have a branch near your home. It is there to provide help and advice for the asking (pp. 99-102).

CHAPTER TWO

The Brain

An epileptic fit has its origin in the brain, and not in the muscles of the limbs or any other part that may become conspicuous during the attack. What then is the connection between the brain and the fit? In order to understand this, we should look a little into the nature and function of the brain itself. The wide variety of types of seizure was referred to in the previous chapter; the frequency, time of occurrence and magnitude of attacks are also important.

Whatever philosophical or theological opinions there may be concerning freedom of thought and action and the ultimate control of the brain, it is clear that it is the organ into which we receive the stimuli that provide experience, and that it is the immediate source of control over our actions. It is the perceptive organ which obtains information from the five senses, and which either stores or rejects it. If stored, this information can be reproduced in the form of memory or may be used to bring about muscular activity, including speech and writing. Actions are, of course, modified, and sometimes determined, by experiences drawn consciously or sub-consciously from the memory store.

The simple input and output mechanism is further influenced by part of the brain concerned with the production of those characteristics which, when added together, create a personality (i.e. that which distinguishes one individual from all others). These include such traits as fear, anxiety, aggression, calmness, or warmth of relationship with other people. Other factors modifying behaviour have to be added to these, such as greed, generosity, and the ability to see another point of view. Considering this, and an infinite number of other variables, one can appreciate the delicacy with which the balance of a pattern of behaviour is constructed.

Behaviour is further modified by the degree of activity of the individual at a particular time. This depends on the rhythm of sleeping and waking, lethargy or alertness, hunger, satiety, or the action of drugs, including alcohol. The experience of pleasure or discomfort, elation or depression, relaxation or tension, will further modify a reaction to a given situation, and this reaction may therefore vary considerably according to different circumstances. This, and much more, is the result of activity in the ten thousand million nerve cells in the brain, which we must now consider in more detail.

Brain structure

A cell is a minute structure, only visible under the microscope, and is the smallest living unit in the body. Cells are the 'bricks' with which the body is constructed. Nerve cells in the brain are connected with one another, and with the remotest parts of the body. They are highly specialised; some concerned with movement being connected eventually to muscles; others concerned with sensation, with the receiving organs which may be in the skin or muscle or a selective mechanism like the ear or eye. Long nerve fibres extending from the cell bodies make these connections, and on reaching its destination, the stimulus, or message may be relayed through several cells (as in the system used to amplify a long-distance telephone call). There are relays in the message systems whether they are travelling to the brain (sensory) or away from it (motor). Other nerve cells modify the message as it passes, in order to influence, for example, the way in which a muscle reacts so that controlled and co-ordinated movements are produced.

There are several ways in which a movement is controlled. The appropriate brain cells responsible for muscle activity (and which are concerned with the movements that may occur during an epileptic fit) are not connected to individual muscle cells; this would require an enormous brain and too complex a mechanism to co-ordinate them. Instead, the motor nerve cells in the brain are concerned with whole movements or actions (e.g. words and their formation) and are connected to all those muscle fibres which are necessary to bring about the entire movement. Other parts of the brain regulate speed and delicacy of action, and act on the impulses initiated by motor nerve cells in order to control them, after the manner of a regulator or governor on a machine. There is also a servo-mechanism, by which a feed-back controls action in accordance with the effect produced.

Between the nerve cells and fibres in the brain and spinal cord, there are other cells (called glia) whose function is to nourish and protect them, and to provide mechanical support, like the soil between the roots of innumerable plants. Incidentally, it is these supporting cells which are the source of the commonest types of brain tumour, which, by irritating the adjacent nerve cells can give rise to epileptic fits in some patients. Nerve cells are darker in colour than glial cells and fibres, so that the cut brain can be seen to consist of grey and white matter according to the predominance of one or the other. The nerve cells (grey matter) form a layer over the folded surface of the brain (cortex) and are also grouped in masses near the centre. In the spinal cord the grey matter (nerve cells) is in the centre and the white matter is around the outside.

Specialised nerve cells are grouped within the brain, so that the function of each of its various parts is more concerned with one activity than another (Fig. 1, p. 8). Nevertheless the brain must not be looked on as a kind of department store in which separate areas have little in common except the name and image of the company. The brain functions as an integrated whole, but can adapt to a certain extent to the removal or destruction of a few of its parts without the effect being very apparent. Individual nerve cells are irreplaceable and are continually falling into disuse throughout life; this is part of the ageing process. They are also extremely susceptible to damage, especially from shortage of oxygen.

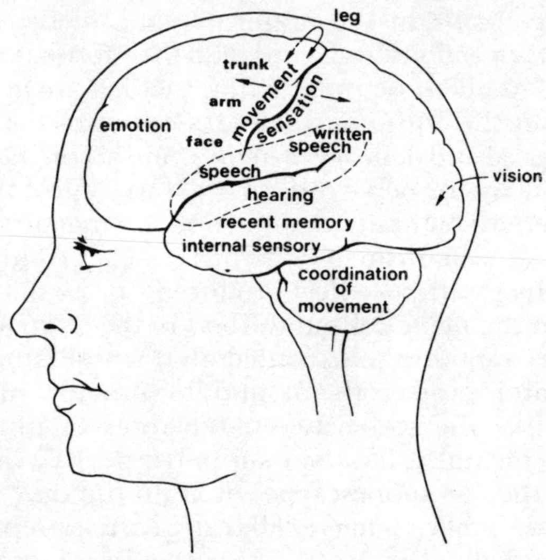

Figure 1   Localisation of function in the dominant half-brain

The complicated inter-activity of nerve cells, which goes on all the time, depends on the precise discharge of minute electrical currents which pass along their nerve fibres when they become active. These currents are produced by chemical changes in and around the cells, and are the sole means by which nerve impulses are transmitted from one place to another. The continuous discharge of millions of these impulses within the brain, and the passage of others through it during both sleeping and waking periods, gives rise to an overall fluctuation in electrical activity or potential; this can be amplified and connected to a recording apparatus so that it vibrates a pen across a moving strip of paper.

These electrical differences may be compared with the hundreds of distinct impulses created by the feet of a column of marching soldiers crossing a bridge, which can produce a rhythm that causes the whole structure to swing and bounce. This rhythm depends on the nature of the bridge itself, together with a complicated mixture of the various impulses which are imparted to it. The rhythm of brain activity is a synthesis of many electrical changes which we can measure by placing electrodes on the scalp, on the surface of the brain, or even within it. The technique of recording these changes is known as electro-encephalography, and the record is familiarly referred to as an EEG or electro-encephalogram.

A moment's reflection will make it clear that these records of the so-called 'brain waves' have fairly well defined limitations and that they only allow the function of the brain to be observed or tested in a very remote way. Unfortunately, only a small part of the brain is accessible, for the electrodes normally have to be placed in relation to an external surface. The underneath aspect of the brain is almost wholly inaccessible and so are the interstices of the folds in the brain itself and the surfaces between its various parts.

The electro-encephalogram

The changes which are recorded in the EEG are the magnified differences in electrical potential – the voltage between two points on the brain. As has been mentioned, these may be recorded through the skull and scalp, or directly from the brain when it is exposed during an operation. Alternatively, the difference in electrical potential between various single points and a 'neutral' reference point (such as the nose), or the average of a number of points, may be compared. The potential differences involved are of the order of 0.001 to 0.005 of a volt, so that considerable amplification is needed. This introduces the possibility of also amplifying other, unwanted changes in electrical potential, such as those arising from muscle and heart action or even from extraneous sources unrelated to the patient.

Rhythmic differences of electrical potential vary according to the part of the brain from which they are picked up. They depend also on the age of the person involved and his mental state; whether he is awake or asleep, concentrating or relaxed, with his eyes open or shut. These rhythms are also affected by many drugs, and by changes in the metabolism or chemical activity within the body.

A flash of bright light produces a stimulus to the brain and causes an alteration of the electrical state. If a brief flash is repeated, it produces an electrical response of the same frequency, which may be great enough to be recorded from the scalp electrodes of the EEG thus imposing a new rhythm on the natural one. This is known as photic stimulation. This may be helpful in detecting the responsiveness of the hinder part of the cerebral hemispheres to demands made upon them. In a susceptible patient, regular stimuli of this nature may so disturb the harmonious electrical activity of the brain as to cause a fit (see p. 19).

An expert can readily distinguish an EEG record taken from a child from that of an adult, and tell if he was asleep or awake (Fig. 2b and c). This is because alterations occur in the shape of the waves and in the patterns of many changes of electrical potential, but despite the numerous ingredients that go to make a single movement of the recording pen, the changes follow recognisable patterns and fit into a stereotype which is often as familiar to the person reading the record as the features which enable one to recognise a well-known face. For instance, a comparison of (a) and (b) in Figure 2 shows an obvious difference, and in (b) there are patterns of tall V-shaped waves not found in the waking record. Although there is a superficial resemblance between the alpha rhythm in (a) and the sleep spindles in (b), careful counting will show that the alpha rhythm in this case has a frequency of eight to nine cycles per second, while that of the sleep spindles is nearly twice as fast. Between the episodes of activity nearly three seconds elapse in which the changes in potential in the brain cells almost cancel each other out and hardly any activity is recorded. The features of the EEG differ according to the depth of sleep, and in dreaming.

In addition to the physiological changes that have been mentioned, and there are many others as well, certain illnesses that affect metabolism may alter the record, for instance, liver failure or diabetes mellitus. Changes induced by the presence of a brain tumour, an abscess, or the scars in the brain following head injury may be used in their detection, although this use of the EEG has been largely superseded by an apparatus which measures X-ray absorption as the beam traverses the brain. This machine (Computerised Axial Tomography or CT scan) produces pictures which are, in effect, pictures of cross-sections of the head, and which reveal the presence of pathology or distortions of the normal anatomy (Fig. 3, p. 15).

The EEG is also changed by disturbance of the blood supply to parts of the brain, and by haemorrhage, but its main use since the advent of CT scanning is in the detection and observation of changes associated with epilepsy in its various forms. Certain types of epilepsy have a recognisable wave pattern. Petit-mal (p. 28), for example, produces characteristic spikes and waves in the trace three times every second. The size and direction of a spike or sharp wave indicates the area of the brain from which a fit may arise, and in grand-mal the generalised disturbance of activity not only confirms the diagnosis but may also sometimes indicate a focal origin (Fig. 4a, p. 23). However, it is important to remember that not all people who have spike forms in their EEG have clinical epilepsy, neither do all people who have fits necessarily have recordable changes in the EEG.

After a brain cell has discharged an impulse there is a brief period during which it is unable to respond because it may be said to be 'recharging'. The electrical discharge from a cell may be compared to one from the sparking plug in the cylinder of an automobile engine. As long as the plugs fire in

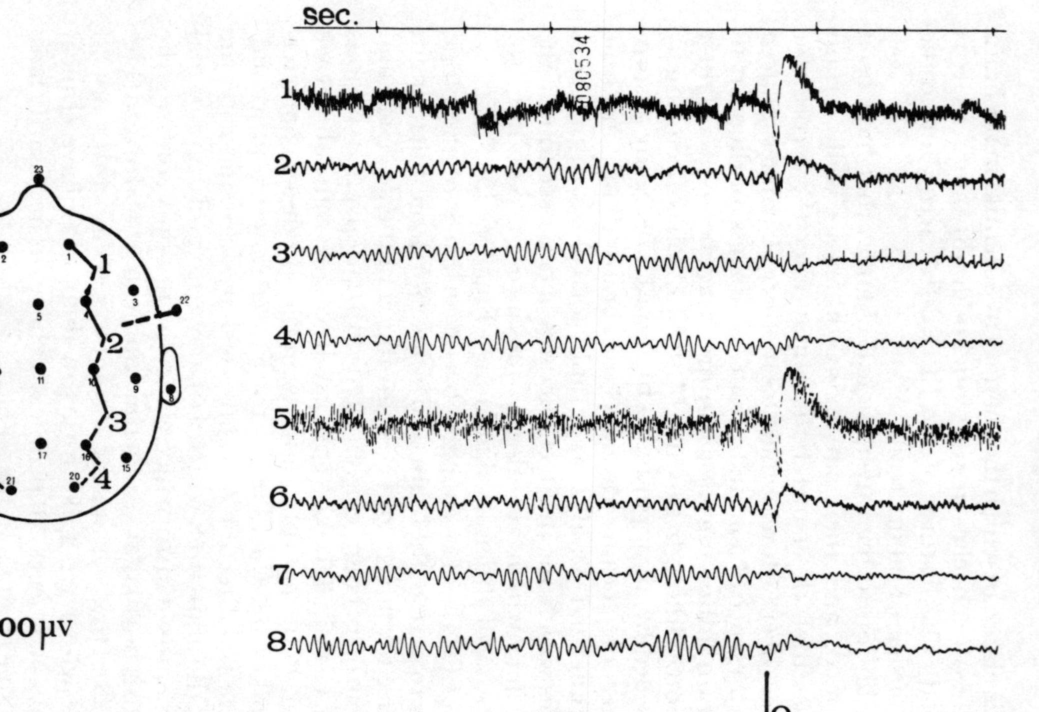

Figure 2 The normal EEG
(a) Trace showing alpha rhythm (8–14 Hz-cycles per second) in all channels except 1 and 5. This is present when the eyes are shut and disappears when they are open (0).

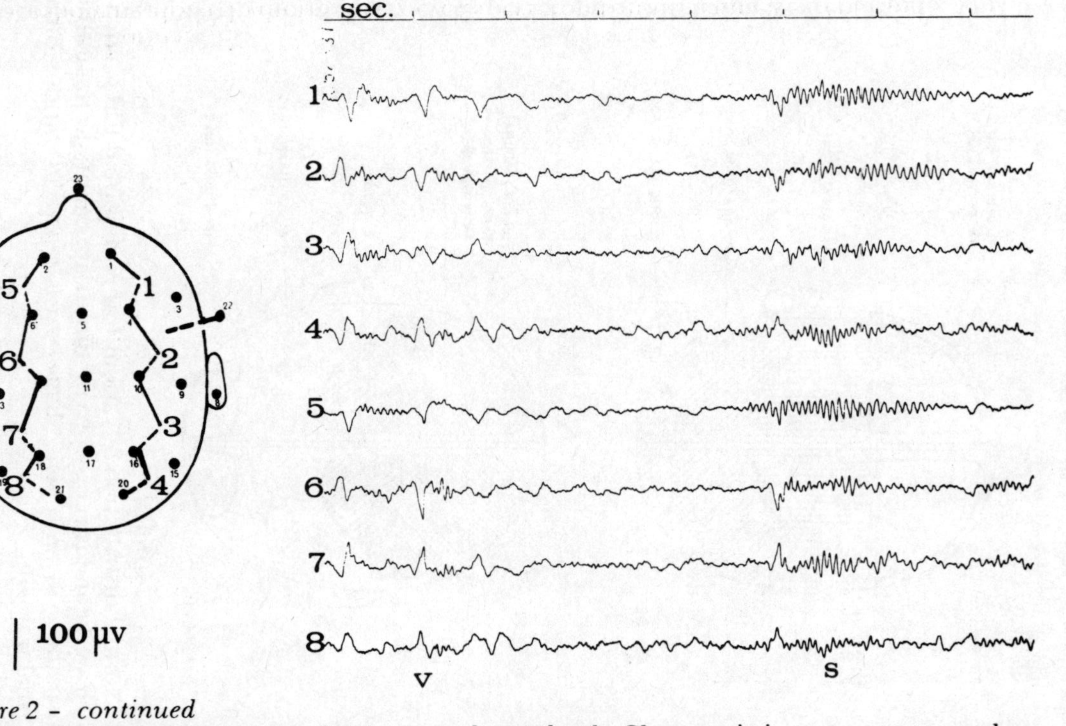

Figure 2 – continued
(b) Trace during normal sleep of light to moderate depth. Characteristic waves are seen at the top of the head (V = vertex) and 'sleep spindles' (S).

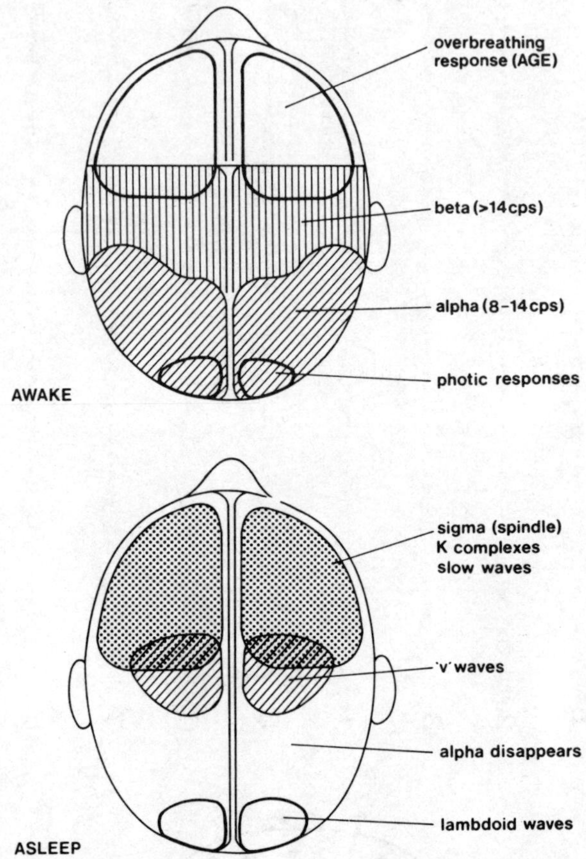

Figure 2 – continued
(c) Normal distribution of various forms of normal EEG activity when awake and asleep. Alpha rhythm disappears in sleep as well as when the eyes are open. Shaded areas represent various other normal waves.

rotation at regular intervals, the pistons will travel up and down evenly, to produce smooth running of the engine. However, if the order of firing is incorrect, or if a plug fires prematurely, the even pattern is interfered with and the engine may hesitate or back-fire. The monotonous hum of the efficient engine is replaced by a disturbing change which may cause anxiety and concern as to what may have gone wrong. Abnormal discharges of nerve cells in the brain disturb the smooth function of the organ in a similar way, and give rise to unwanted activity or prevent wanted activity, or both. This is the basis of an epileptic fit. Disturbances of activity in nerve cells may be self-perpetuating, like a chain reaction, so that abnormal behaviour of relatively few cells may build up an influence over many others to which they are connected. If these are then brought into activity in a disorderly manner, they can no longer function properly for their true purpose, so that eventually the function of the brain as a whole may be disturbed.

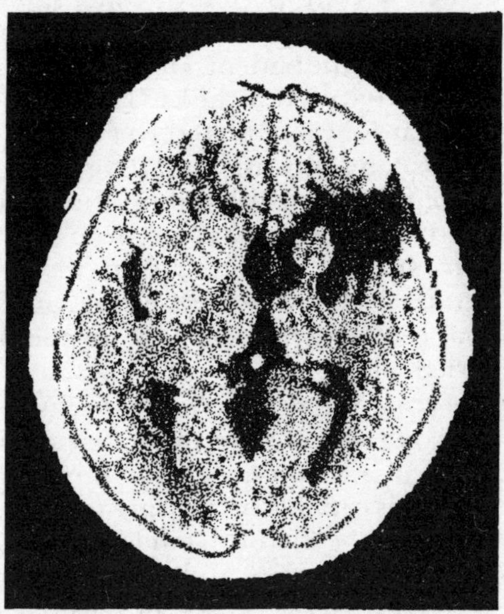

Figure 3   Computerised Axial Tomography (CT scan)
In the right upper quadrant a dark area in the brain represents an area of brain damage which was the source of epilepsy. Other darker areas are the ventricles or normal brain cavities.

In order to make an abnormal wave pattern more obvious it may be necessary to record during sleep, whether natural or produced by a sedative, or to change the chemistry of the blood by rapid breathing. Very occasionally a fit may be induced so that it can be observed and recorded and the correct treatment given. This may be done by withdrawing anticonvulsant tablets (which may bring out an epileptic focus in the EEG without inducing a seizure) or by the administration of certain drugs. Other substances produce their own effects on the EEG, and brain function can be assessed by studying these. Needle electrodes are sometimes placed below the brain by introducing them in front of the ear, and this enables activity to be recorded from areas that are not accessible on the surface. Even more unusually, a record may be made over a long period of time, say twenty-four hours, by connecting the scalp electrodes to a small transmitter attached to the patient. He may then eat, sleep and continue normal activity while the EEG is picked up within a radius of several yards by a radio receiver which records it on magnetic tape for later scrutiny and diagnosis. Sometimes records are made from leads placed on the brain surface at operation (electro-corticography) or from wire electrodes introduced into specific nuclei within the brain (depth electrodes). These sophisticated techniques are only undertaken in special centres where surgery for the treatment of epilepsy is carried out.

The nature of epileptic attacks will be discussed in detail in the next chapter; but already we can see that a dysfunction of this kind can occur in anyone, in the same way that any automobile engine is capable of running irregularly or back-firing. Fortunately, the natural tendency of the brain is towards harmonious function, and normally a considerable disturbance is required to upset it. However, in some individuals disharmony can be more easily produced than in others. It has been said that we are all 'epileptics', for any of us can suffer a seizure if the appropriate circumstances arise. This is a good reason for not using the word 'epileptic' to describe an individual who has fits, for the only thing which distinguishes him from other people is the fact that the *threshold* at which his seizures occur is lower than in the average person. Furthermore, this threshold may vary from time to time and in different parts of the brain, so that the smooth functioning of one small area may be more readily disturbed than that of other parts; such an area becomes a focus of abnormal activity – which may result in a focal fit affecting that specific part of the brain – and this may spread to involve progressively other parts of the grey matter perhaps ending in a generalised fit or a succession of them. The nature of a seizure therefore depends very much on the function of the area of the brain that is affected by abnormal electrical activity at the onset of the attack and thereafter. The electrical activity, which we can measure and record, is itself the product of chemical changes inside and outside the brain cells. Thus the chemistry of the body and that of the drugs used to treat epilepsy are intimately related to the events described in the next chapter.

CHAPTER THREE

Epileptic Fits

As we saw in Chapter 2, the orderly firing of impulses from the nerve cells in the brain can be recorded as changes in electrical potential which vary according to the age of the patient, and between his sleeping and waking states. However, there are some wave forms which are peculiarly characteristic of epilepsy, and their nature and frequency may be very important in diagnosis. One of the most characteristic features is a short, relatively high-voltage impulse generally known as a 'spike'. The appearance of these spikes in a record may enable the location of an abnormality to be determined.

While spikes show which part of the brain is the source of abnormal discharges (which may be revealed as an epileptic seizure), this may not necessarily be the exact situation of the source of the irritation. It is more likely that a scar or tumour will give rise to abnormal discharges around its borders than that a discharge should arise within the abnormal area itself. By tracing the location of abnormal discharges doctors can identify a pathological area and sometimes determine whether it is possible to remove it (Fig. 4a, p. 23). However, not everyone with spike forms in his or her EEG is subject to epilepsy, much as this may indicate susceptibility to the condition; nor does everyone who has epilepsy produce this type of record. The EEG is therefore a poor guide to the probability of epilepsy occurring in any given guide to the fact which is especially important in connection with legal problems following a head injury. Often one rhythm or pattern is superimposed upon another, and this may make interpretation quite difficult. Certain drugs affect the frequency of the normal brain voltage rhythm and the changes induced by these drugs may be used as a means of making an abnormality more obvious.

Changes in the blood chemistry, particularly that of the blood sugar, may also alter the electrical activity of the brain. In people who have a low epileptic threshold, this may mean that a low blood sugar level produces a state in which fits are more liable to occur. Shortage of oxygen as a result of exertion, choking or altitude increases the liability to attacks, as does tiredness, fear or anger.

Any abnormal discharge from a brain cell may be the source of other discharges, which may sufficiently disorganise the function of the brain as a whole for it to be noticeable by the individual concerned or by others. However, it is important to recognise that in the same way that epilepsy is a symptom of an abnormality in the brain, the electrical changes are also brought about by the abnormality, and they do not constitute the primary change which is probably chemical. Enough has been said to show that fits of any kind have a purely physical basis even if its exact nature is not completely known, and they are not the product of any abnormality of the mind. This point will be enlarged on in the next chapter.

Localisation of function in the brain

The main source of impulses controlling movement lies in a strip of brain surface (cortex) running obliquely downwards and forwards from a point just behind the centre of the top of the head (see Fig. 1, p. 8). The cells in this strip are arranged in an orderly fashion so that those which control the lower limbs are at the top, and those which control the arms, hands and face are at the bottom.

The two sides of the brain do not function in exactly the same way, for not only are they related to the opposite sides of the body, but one side governs more powerful and controllable movement, which gives rise to right or left handedness. In most people, one half of the brain is dominant in this way, and contains the areas which are responsible for speech and associated functions such as writing and reading.

When this part of the brain does not work properly, as is sometimes the case after an epileptic fit, a person may be fully conscious and aware of his surroundings, knowing what to say, but unable to form words or letters, and thus unable to communicate. He may also be fully alert, but temporarily unable to understand words, commands, or writing, until the affected cells begin to function again. This lingering loss of function after a fit (sometimes referred to as Todd's paralysis) may also produce temporary paralysis or weakness if any of the cells controlling movement are involved.

Behind the movement area is the region of the brain concerned with appreciation of the position of the parts of the body and other forms of sensation. At the extreme hinder end of the brain is the main area for appreciation of sight. Fits more commonly arise from the front and middle areas of the brain than from the back.

The temporal lobes, which are found in the lower third of the cerebral hemispheres are responsible for appreciation of internal information from the abdominal organs and from the senses of smell and hearing. They are also intimately concerned with the memory of recent events, which is subsequently passed on elsewhere for more permanent retention.

The diagram (Fig. 1, p. 8) must be regarded as a general guide to localisation and no more. Imagine viewing Europe from a satellite, from which one assumes that most Frenchmen are in France, and most Spaniards in Spain, though not all of them are to be found exclusively in these two places. So it is with the brain; the boundaries of function are only rough guides to how the brain controls activities and behaviour.

Types of seizure, fits or epilepsy

Focal epilepsy
It is possible for a few cells in the motor or movement area to

send stimuli to a muscle in the face or elsewhere and cause a twitch, even though there is no voluntary motivation. After this the cells may function normally again. Even such an inconspicuous event as this may fall into the category of a minor seizure for it was an involuntary, uncontrolled action. In this example it would be called a *focal fit* because it had an epileptogenic focus in a particular and recognisable area of the brain (Fig. 4a, p. 23). There would be no interference with thought or consciousness, provided the changes were confined to that particular area. The EEG would probably show a spike over the lower part of the motor cortex which is concerned with facial movement, for example, if one were able to make a record when it was happening. Activity of this type is seen in Figure 4a but the focus in that particular case is in the temporal lobe, slightly lower in the brain than the area of face representation.

However, there are other possibilities; the abnormal discharges may affect adjacent cells, causing the attack to spread along the strip of brain concerned with movement so that the muscle twitches affect the hand, arm, shoulder or whatever part of the brain is stimulated in this way. When a focal fit spreads in this manner, it is named *Jacksonian epilepsy*, after Hughlings Jackson, who first described it scientifically in the nineteenth century.

This type of fit may remain confined to the muscles which were first affected, and die out without anything else happening. Sometimes, it may continue to spread and involve other areas of the brain, including those central structures which are concerned with consciousness and awareness. The result is that the patient becomes unconscious (and may fall to the ground) until the situation returns to normal. The duration of each step in the development of the attack may be brief or last for several minutes. The widespread involvement of the brain just described is likely to cause a major seizure or grand-mal attack.

The grand-mal or major seizure
There is another type of seizure which, instead of starting on

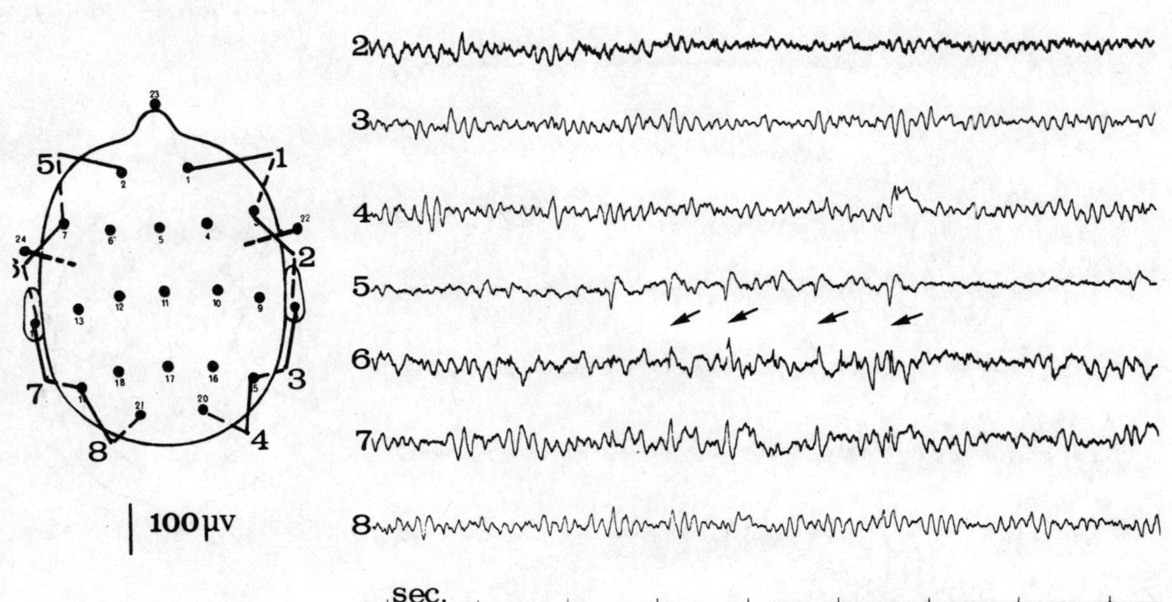

Figure 4 The abnormal EEG
(a) Trace showing spike forms from the left side of the brain. The spikes seen in channels 5 and 6 point towards each other because their source lies near the electrode common to these two channels.

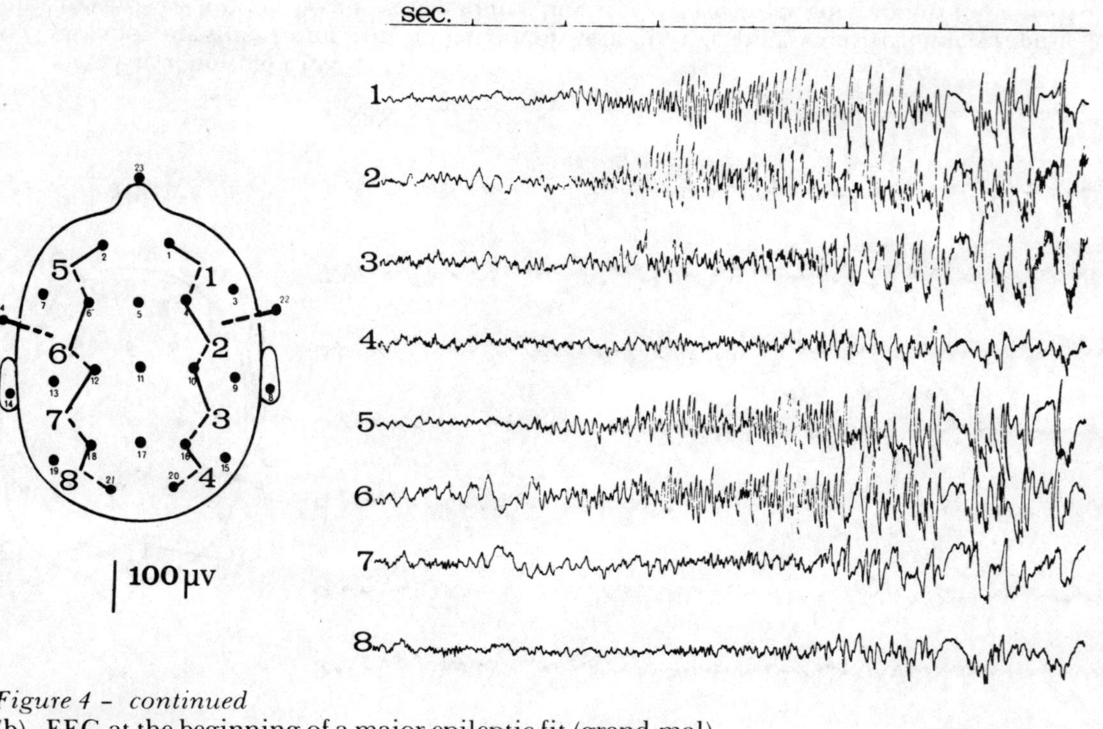

Figure 4 – continued
(b) EEG at the beginning of a major epileptic fit (grand-mal).

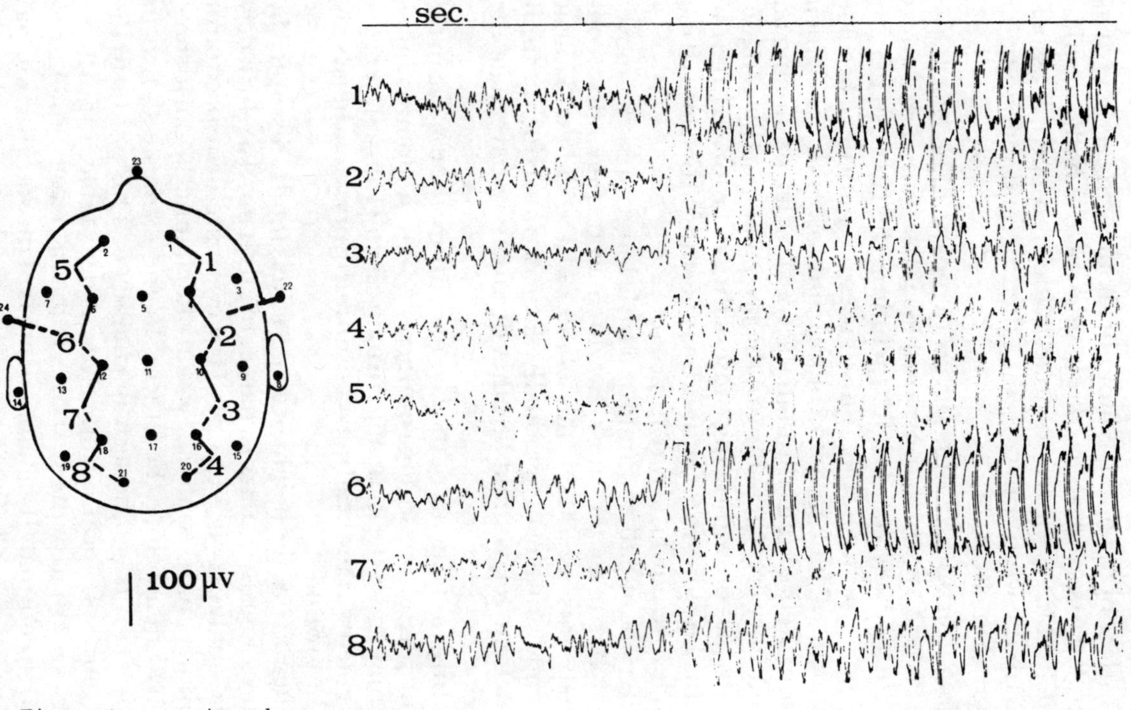

Figure 4 – continued
(c) EEG in petit-mal. Spike and wave forms occur almost equally in all channels at the onset of the attack.

the surface of the brain, is brought about by the activity of its central parts, and affects both sides of the body simultaneously. This is the type of attack which most people associate with the word epilepsy. It is called a grand-mal or major seizure (Fig. 4b, p. 24).

Characteristically, this fit has two parts. The first is the *tonic phase,* in which consciousness is lost, muscles contract and the body becomes rigid, including the chest, so that air does not enter the lungs. This causes the patient to become cyanosed, or blue-grey in colour, and forces the air which remains in the lungs through the vocal cords, producing an involuntary cry. Clenching of the jaws may trap the tongue, and absence of swallowing causes saliva to be forced from the mouth. The limbs are rigid and may be straight or bent. All the muscles are powerfully contracted.

After about half a minute or a little longer, jerking movements begin in the muscles which were previously contracted; this is called the *clonic phase.* These violent rhythmic movements gradually decrease in frequency until the patient relaxes and breathes deeply to re-oxygenate the blood.

Biting movements of the jaw may injure the tongue in the clonic phase, and strong contraction of the abdominal muscles may cause the patient to urinate or soil himself. Jerking movements of the head may cause him injury when he is lying on the ground.

The EEG at the height of a major fit is totally disrupted by high voltage irregular discharges in all channels, which defy visual analysis (Fig. 4b, p. 24). However, careful inspection or computer analysis may show that one channel began to show dysrhythmia before the others. In the example shown in Figure 4a this can be seen in channel 6. This points to the possibility of a focal, but otherwise undetectable, origin to the attack. Similarly, the first affected area may be the last to return to normal. If a major seizure is of the so-called idiopathic variety, in which no superficial focal origin occurs, the evidence of the attack is likely to appear simultaneously in all the scalp leads, since the source of the fit lies in the deep central brain structures.

At the end of the attack the exhausted sufferer may pass from a state of unconsciousness, due to the seizure, into a deep sleep. This may be quite brief, or he may not wake for an hour or two. He may well have a headache on waking. If he does not sleep he is likely to be confused on regaining consciousness after the attack, as he gradually becomes aware of what has happened and where he is, rather like the brief disorientation experienced on waking out of a deep sleep in unfamiliar surroundings.

If an epileptic attack is seen to be happening, it is extremely important to note every detail of what takes place. In this way the pattern of development of the fit can be recognised, in the hope of identifying the part of the brain from which the seizure arose. This applies to attacks of any kind. Focal attacks may abort or continue in the same pattern (epilepsia partialis continuans), or turn into grand-mal. In such cases consciousness may not be lost until the head is involved or the fit becomes generalised.

At the onset of a focal fit or other seizure, the patient may experience a feeling of being ill at ease, or have a sensation or movement somewhere, which is a warning to him that an attack is about to begin. Some warnings may not develop into a full attack. Some sufferers can abort their seizure by some useful trick, such as restraining the movement of an arm, or concentrating hard on something as soon as the warning occurs. Any form of warning or *aura* represents the very beginning of a seizure. The length of time between the aura and the next part of the fit may be enough to allow precautions to be taken, such as moving to a safer place, sitting down or removing dentures. On the other hand, the warning period may be too brief to be of any value in this respect. Drug treatment may affect the aura. This is important if it causes it to disappear. Because the aura is the beginning of the fit, changes will occur in the EEG while it is taking place, and these may be focal or generalised.

Petit-mal

There are yet other varieties of epilepsy, such as the brief attacks which affect young people between the ages of five and twelve years and are known as *petit-mal*. This is a specific type of fit and must not be confused with minor epilepsy, which is as much as anything a description of the magnitude of a seizure. Unfortunately the term is very loosely used, often by people who should know better.

In true petit-mal there is a brief lapse of consciousness of which the patient, and even those with him, may be unaware. A momentary change of colour in the face (usually pallor), a pause in the conversation, a movement of the eyelids or a slight jerk of a limb may be all that is visible. The EEG has a characteristic pattern during the attack, in which a slow wave lasting about a third of a second is followed by a sharp spike, with a frequency of about three complexes a second (Fig. 4c, p. 25). Sometimes the attack may occur without anything being noticed by the patient, his teacher or any other observer.

If attacks occur very frequently – and they may take place many times in an hour – the performance of a child at school may be seriously impaired; control of them will then bring about an apparent increase in alertness and skill in performance and learning. Brief 'absences' occur in other forms of epilepsy and have a superficial resemblance to petit-mal, but they do not have the specific EEG changes necessary for the diagnosis. The distinction is very important, for it will be seen, when we consider the treatment of epilepsy, that petit-mal will respond to certain drugs which are inappropriate in other forms of seizure (see p. 47).

Temporal lobe epilepsy

Another type of focal epilepsy is of special importance. This involves the temporal lobes, which are found in the lower third of the main part of the brain (cerebral hemisphere) on either side. This large area is connected to many central nerve cells and is concerned with memory (see p. 21), the senses of smell and hearing, and awareness of one's 'insides'.

The auras of attacks arising in this situation are varied and often dramatic. They may take the form of a hallucination of sight, sound, or a sense of unfamiliarity in a well-known place. Objects may appear large or small in an *Alice in Wonderland* manner, the world may seem unreal, or the individual no longer himself. Fear or anger may accompany or be part of the aura, occasionally leading to aggressive behaviour which the patient cannot voluntarily control, and of which he may not subsequently be aware. Sometimes there is an indescribable feeling in the head or stomach.

These attacks are known as *temporal lobe* or *psychomotor* seizures. Their variety is so great that the appearance to an on-looker cannot easily be described. The first signs may be a change in skin colour and turning of the head and eyes in one direction. During a fit chewing movements may occur or a stereotyped irrelevant phrase may be uttered. Semi-purposeful movements, for example, smoothing the hair or straightening the tie may take place; sometimes even an article of clothing may be removed. Although he may appear dazed during the attack, it is possible for a person having a fit to seem to others to be in possession of his faculties and yet he himself does not know what is happening. Very occasionally the fit may be associated with violent behaviour, but only when this is a regular feature of the fit-pattern. In such cases, of course, the individual is quite unaware of what he is doing, and has no memory of what may have happened when consciousness has been regained.

The attack may turn into a grand-mal seizure, or it may end with groping in the air as if the sufferer were searching for something or trying to find his whereabouts by peering in various directions. Occasionally the end of the attack is hard to recognise because a person may start behaving in a seemingly rational, but entirely automatic way, and in this state actions are not determined by his will but follow one upon another as if by habit. During a period of automatism the patient with epilepsy may undertake a complicated journey, asking for directions and buying tickets, threading his way through traffic, and continuing to do so for periods of half an hour or less, or for several hours. Yet he may appear completely normal to everyone who sees him. At the end of the episode he will, of course, not know how he came to be where he is and may even be lost. However, behaviour of this kind is rare. Usually actions during an attack follow the natural pattern of the sufferer's life, with no behaviour occurring in the dream state that is alien to his character.

Status epilepticus and serial seizures
When epilepsy is poorly controlled, or occasionally for other reasons, one fit may be succeeded by another after a brief interval. It is important that successive attacks should be brought to an end as soon as possible; medical help is usually necessary for this, particularly if there is no pause between attacks – a condition known as *status epilepticus* which can cause serious damage to the brain or be fatal (unlike the majority of seizures, from which the patient generally recovers spontaneously and without harm).

It is imperative that medical aid is summoned urgently to any patient with status epilepticus. Focal attacks involving little movement and no loss of consciousness are less of an emergency if they continue one after another. Rarely is it necessary to call a doctor or to send a patient to hospital after an isolated minor seizure.

Childhood seizures
Some types of fit are unique to childhood. Take for instance the so-called salaam attack, in which an infant may bend forward abruptly for a moment; like petit-mal this has a characteristic EEG pattern. There are other attacks consisting of sudden muscular jerks or episodes of stiffness, and attacks may be precipitated by breath-holding. In principle, however, the abnormalities of cerebral activity are similar to those in adults. However, the importance of preventing attacks, and especially serial seizures or status epilepticus is even greater. The reason is that the young brain is easily

damaged by lack of oxygen during fits, and possibly by other factors, and injury to the brain cells resulting from childhood convulsions may produce seizures in later life, particularly those of the temporal lobe variety.

In some young children seizures are easily induced by a rise in body temperature incidental to an illness such as measles or gastro-enteritis. A single episode of 'febrile convulsions' or 'teething convulsions' need not necessarily be of dire significance for the future, but it should never be ignored. The best way to prevent recurrence is usually to take steps to control fever with aspirin or external cooling. Febrile convulsions indicate a susceptibility to attacks, but more important than this, a series of them may so damage the brain as to cause epileptic seizures later, as has been mentioned. In Copenhagen an emergency 'flying squad' has been set up specially to treat childhood seizures, a measure which, though not possible as a universal policy, underlines the seriousness of repeated attacks in this age group.

About 75 per cent of all those people who will develop epilepsy will have had their first fit by the age of eight years. Indeed, the first seizure is more likely to happen during the first two years of life than during any subsequent period. As the child becomes older many of those who had seizures when they were very young will have 'grown out of them', and be free of their disability.

As in older age groups, attacks in children may be related to an inherited low threshold (p.32), but they may also derive from certain hereditary disorders of the skin and nervous tissues or from various metabolic disorders. Seizures may be associated with maldevelopment of the brain or with infections that may or may not have shown a clear clinical picture of meningitis or encephalitis. Injury is a common cause of epilepsy at any age, but particularly in childhood and infancy. Indeed, it may occur during the process of birth. Most of the causative factors which operate in adults are also important in the diagnosis of childhood epilepsy.

Incidence of attacks

About a half of all epileptic attacks are of grand-mal, or major type, though some may start in a focal manner. A third are of the temporal lobe type and may occasionally become major. Any individual may have both major and some other form of attack but whether there is one variety or several, they remain remarkably consistent for that particular person. Indeed, a change in the type of attack may be of importance and should be reported to whoever is caring for the patient.

Although epilepsy begins most frequently in the young, there is another peak time of onset, namely during the years of puberty and adolescence, and again much later among the elderly. Almost all those who will suffer from epilepsy, except when it is due to acquired disease or injury, will have had their first attack by the age of twenty.

Threshold of epilepsy and the acquisition of attacks

We saw earlier (p. 17) that the manifestation of epilepsy depends on the *threshold* at which activity of the nerve cells becomes disorganised. This threshold is determined to some extent by inheritance, but it is no more than a degree of susceptibility which is passed on, and not the fits themselves. Stringent laws against marriage between those who have had fits, which used to exist in some countries, were founded on a misunderstanding. Clearly, the chances of a child having a low epileptic threshold are greater if the mother and father are both subject to fits, but if one parent has a high or normal threshold and the other has a low one, the chances of epilepsy appearing in their children are not great unless some potent cause, such as a head injury, supervenes (see also p. 31).

Damage to the brain during birth is a common cause of epilepsy and it is, to some extent, preventable. Focal fits may follow damage to the cells on the surface layers of the brain, and may cause other types of seizure.

Damaged brain cells as a result of infection or fever can also give rise to seizures. Tumours of the brain, and certain abnormalities of development can irritate neighbouring cells in one way or another with the same result. Epilepsy can therefore be acquired as a result of injury or disease at any time of life. Damage to the brain from an injury, whatever the cause, provided it is of sufficient severity, can leave a scar capable of causing irritation in the neighbourhood. If an early fit is associated with a head injury, penetration of the brain by a spike of bone or a foreign body, or prolonged confusion of mind, the chances of subsequent epilepsy are sufficiently great to make many doctors prescribe anti-convulsant drugs as an insurance against having an attack, even if one did not occur immediately after the injury. However, this is only a safeguard and not a guarantee of immunity.

Operations on some areas of the brain may produce a risk of fits, and similar precautions may be necessary. Of course, many of the conditions for which brain operations are per-formed are themselves productive of attacks. It must be remem-bered that none of us is exempt from any of these possibilities.

Certain factors can make attacks more likely to occur; some of these may be related to the individual, such as the amount of sugar in the blood, the phase of the menstrual cycle or pregnancy in women, or the emotional state. Other factors are environmental and include, for example, triggering by a mental shock such as might follow the news of an unexpected death, or by a sudden flash of temper. This is what happened when someone who had difficulty in seeing to her left side accidentally bumped into a passer-by in the street and was accused of being drunk. The injustice of the situation caused her to become angry and this in turn precipitated an attack. She also suffered a fit brought on by fear when she heard burglars entering a neighbouring flat which she knew to be unoccupied.

Another patient, who had sustained a head injury two or three months previously, had to get up early to catch a plane. He only just managed to get to the airport on time but had no time for breakfast. He did not eat or drink on the short flight, and on arrival he took a taxi straight to an appointment. Shortly afterwards he had his first seizure, precipitated in his case by a low blood sugar level through lack of food.

A few people have their attacks brought on by listening to music, by loud noises, or even by reading. Alcohol, too, increases any susceptibility to attacks as do a variety of chemicals and chronic poisons, such as lead. Certain drugs are known to produce attacks, and may even deliberately be used for this purpose if it is necessary to examine a fit in detail before considering an operation to remove the part of the brain that is the source of the trouble.

The best known external precipitating factor is a flashing source of light. However, it appears that these flashes have to impinge directly on the eyes from the front, and not from the side, so the stimuli from the sun shining through a row of poplars beside the road may precipitate an attack by throwing bright patches of reflection on the road surface rather than from light in the gaps which may be seen between the trees. Some people get fits if they gaze at flashing signals on a television set, and anyone liable to this kind of attack should not stand in front of the set to adjust it. However, both these sources of seizures are probably much less important than used to be thought.

The time of day is also significant, for there are differences in the chemistry of the body over a twenty-four-hour period, some of which may influence the time when attacks occur. It is not uncommon for attacks to take place at night and never in the daytime, a fact that may be a very important consideration when it comes, for example, to assessing eligibility to hold a driving licence (p. 80).

Finally, it is worth mentioning the risk of acquiring parasites from animals, which may settle in the brain and cause fits. Cysticercosis, which is caused by a parasite which lives on sheep and other animals not normally domesticated, constitutes a negligible risk in urban populations, but dogs may carry toxicaris. In ordinary circumstances, the risk of picking up the infestation is very small, but children who take their pets to bed with them are increasing the chances of doing so to a significant extent, so this attractive but potentially harmful practice should be strongly discouraged.

CHAPTER FOUR

Associated Disorders and Causes of Fits

In many cases, the cause or even the precipitating factor which brings about epileptic fits is not known, which has led to their being labelled 'idiopathic' or of unknown origin. As we learn more about the susceptibility of the brain to certain diseases and changes in the chemistry of the blood, more reasons for the occurrence of epilepsy are being discovered. The condition may not show itself for many years after the causal event. This emphasises the point that epilepsy is a symptom of brain malfunction and not a disease in its own right. It is no more than the manifestation of disordered discharges of electrical activity from certain brain cells.

When brain damage results from injury to the head at birth, or from infection, lack of oxygen, the effects of poisons, the results of head injury in later life, or the presence of tumours, there may be permanent impairment of function in the affected part of the brain. Epilepsy may or may not follow, depending on where the injury was sustained and many other things, some of which were mentioned in Chapter 2 (see *threshold*, p. 17).

Following a fit there may also be transient impairment of function, and this may reveal a hitherto hidden disability. Thus doctors commonly find that a child who is paralysed on one side as a result of damage to the opposite side of the brain, also suffers from focal and possibly generalised fits. Added weakness after a fit may make a minor paralysis more obvious.

If a patient has had a skull fracture, as a result of which some bone fragments were driven inwards and damaged the surface of the brain in the area concerned with speech, he may have permanent difficulty in finding words or in reading and writing, or this may be a symptom which only appears from time to time. In fact, this may be a means whereby the origin of an attack can be determined.

Clearly, the amount of brain damage resulting from any of the factors referred to above may be sufficient to impair general intellectual and emotional behaviour. The disability of epilepsy can be an additional burden. On the other hand, even the occasional occurrence of a fit may interfere with the education of a child who is intellectually normal, or it may prevent an adult from marrying or obtaining employment. It is therefore extremely important that attacks should be as effectively treated as possible and that they should be viewed sympathetically. Some people - mercifully fewer and fewer - still equate epilepsy with stupidity, a misconception that is clearly shown up by the existence of many highly intelligent sufferers. Nevertheless, epilepsy *does* occur in association with some conditions in which the brain is undoubtedly functioning imperfectly, and these conditions bias attitudes generally towards people with epilepsy. If attacks occur at frequent intervals or if they are severe they may damage the brain further, so that if they cannot be prevented altogether or at least reduced in frequency, physical and intellectual performance will often decline. Some of the drugs which are used in the control of epilepsy may themselves have deleterious side-effects on ability or awareness. This has to be balanced against their effectiveness in controlling attacks.

Brain damage apart, the vast majority of patients with epilepsy have normal intelligence and mental faculties, and in most of them the attacks are completely or almost completely controlled. Only one in ten children with epilepsy and no other handicap has to be educated in a special school of one sort or another, while the remainder are able to fit into the normal educational system. Of the ten per cent for whom special educational facilities are needed only a tiny fraction are at residential schools because of their epilepsy. The remainder are educationally subnormal because of some associated disorder, in which epilepsy is an incidental problem.

Epilepsy, personality and emotions

Confusion between idiopathic and acquired forms of epilepsy, and those conditions described above in which epilepsy is incidental to some other major disorder, has led many people to the misguided notion that there is some kind of 'personality' which is peculiar to people with epilepsy. They will call on such folk wisdom as 'you only had to look at him to know he suffered from fits', without any logical justification. Research shows that there is no such thing as an 'epileptic personality'; people with epilepsy share all the characteristics and personality traits of the rest of the population. However, if an individual experiences any handicap in childhood, is shunned by society, is prevented from using his intellectual powers and, above all, is constantly reminded that he is different from the majority, he may well feel that everyone is against him and become depressed, resentful and withdrawn. He may even think of suicide. This is the real nature of the 'epileptic personality'.

Crime and epilepsy

Violent and irrational behaviour contrary to the sufferer's true nature occasionally occurs during an epileptic attack, particularly in association with those of temporal type, though this is not likely to happen as an isolated event in someone whose seizures have in the past been non-aggressive. As a rule, attacks associated with violence are very rare. When they do occur in individual cases, they can often be anticipated. Patients with problems of this nature are usually under continuous medical care, and they are unlikely to seek employment unless attacks are very rare. Adequate medical treatment may prevent episodes of this nature taking place.

A study of the incidence of crimes of violence in a group of prisoners not suffering from epilepsy showed that 22 per cent of them had a history of violent crime. By contrast, the incidence among prisoners who did have epilepsy was 15 per cent. People with epilepsy are not more likely to be violent and aggressive than the rest of the population.

On a more general level the incidence of criminal acts among patients with epilepsy is no greater than among the population as a whole. Epilepsy and crime may be linked or rather correlated. After all, it is not surprising that an individual of low intelligence and subject to depression, who may also bear a grudge, because of his condition, is tempted to get his own back on society one way or another. However, this is quite different from saying that epilepsy is a direct *cause* of anti-social or criminal behaviour.

Most crimes require careful planning and without this strategy they are not likely to succeed. This alone explains why crimes are very rarely carried out during a fit and without the volition of the individual. Indeed, if a habitual criminal carries out a crime during a fit, he is very likely to be caught. This happened to a 'professional' burglar who was caught by the police, sitting on the doorstep of the house he had recently burgled, without his gloves, and having returned to the scene of a previous crime. He carried out the robbery during a period of 'automatic' behaviour following a fit and was believed when he denied any memory of it.

CHAPTER FIVE

What to Do – General Principles and Some Notes on Treatment

When seizures are very brief there may not be time to come to the help of a patient, nor is any assistance necessarily required. If it looks as if the person having a fit may sink to the ground or fall, a helping hand for a moment of support may suffice. In any circumstances, if it looks as if the patient may harm himself he should be firmly but gently directed away from the source of injury, or a dangerous object may be removed. Any physical restraint needed should be firm but coaxing, rather than violent and restricting. Rough treatment is likely to provoke an aggressive response, as it would in any other person who was awakened from sleep to find someone pinning him down by his arms and legs.

Epileptic attacks are very seldom fatal, even though the sufferer sometimes looks extremely ill. This can be frightening to someone seeing a major seizure for the first time, but provided the patient does not harm himself and the attack is not followed by others, he is likely to wake up in due course, as he will have done on many previous occasions.

Sufferers from epilepsy are liable to harm in a wide variety of circumstances. These should be taken into account when considering employment or involvement in sporting or school activities (see Chapters 6, 7 and 8).

The individual or his relatives are likely to be aware of situations in which harm may occur, but should also be alert to the dangers of over-protection. Excessive caution on the part of anxious parents may ruin the life of a young person if overdone. It is essential to allow the sufferer to lead as normal a life as possible, so that any necessary restrictions can be as unobtrusive as is compatible with safety. Regulations on driving are referred to in Chapter 9.

First aid for epilepsy

Everybody should know how to react to a situation in which someone has a major seizure or grand-mal attack, one of the basic conditions requiring first aid. It is likely to be encountered more often than the need to administer artificial respiration for drowning.

The first essential is to act calmly and prevent panic among other people. Because the fit will have to be allowed to take its course, action has to be of a protective nature. Clothing should be loosened around the neck. If the mouth is open, a knotted handkerchief can be placed between the teeth in order to stop the person biting his tongue. However, one should try not to force the mouth open in order to introduce something between the teeth, and care must be taken not to obstruct the passage of air, or to allow one's own fingers to get in the mouth.

If the situation in which the patient is lying is dangerous, he should be moved. If he is in the tonic (rigid) stage of the attack, one must not be surprised when the clonic (rhythmic or jerking) movements begin; and these may make it difficult to reposition him. If possible, the patient should lie on his side rather than on his back which may cause him to choke. If a soft object such as a coat is available, it should be placed beneath the head in order to prevent injury from banging the head on the ground.

When the attack is over there is usually no need to call a doctor or to send the patient to hospital, unless there is a succession of attacks. The patient may be temporarily confused and complain of headache, and in these circumstances should be allowed to sit or lie quietly (in a protected situation) until he feels better.

It is very important not to give the patient anything to drink until he is fully conscious. He may carry a card issued by the British Epilepsy Association, or a wrist strap or disc on a neck chain (Medicalert), saying what should be done, what drugs he takes, how long the fit usually lasts, and who, if anyone, should be contacted. If the patient sleeps after an attack he should be allowed to do so if this is possible, though clearly it may not always be convenient. It is essential to be sure that he is no longer confused or behaving irrationally when he is allowed to go his own way; in other words, make sure the fit is over. If there is any doubt, go with him.

As people get older their fits tend to become less frequent, and often cease altogether. Whether this happens or not depends to some extent on the age of onset, and on the nature of the underlying condition, if any, where epilepsy is merely one of a number of symptoms. In the case of the particular form of epilepsy known as petit-mal (NB: not minor epilepsy, but the type associated with three or four per second spike and wave complexes in the EEG, see p. 28) the brief episodes of disturbed consciousness usually cease by about twenty years of age, though they may be replaced by attacks of another type. On the other hand, epilepsy may be a symptom of some other disorder when it appears for the first time in an older person and should be carefully investigated.

Until attacks have ceased for several years, it is necessary to prevent or control them by the use of drugs. Occasionally the cause of fits can be identified and removed by surgery, but this is seldom possible; in the majority of patients fits have to be controlled or prevented by medication.

Treatment of epilepsy by medicines

If medicines are prescribed it is essential that they are taken regularly. Nothing should be allowed to interfere with this; suddenly omitting to take tablets can be a powerful precipitating cause of attacks. If it is inconvenient to take a mid-day dose, rather than omit it altogether, a patient should ask if the times of his medication can be changed. Some drugs are used up slowly and can be given at long intervals, while others are used up quickly and need to be replaced if an even concentration in the blood is to be maintained.

It is a good idea to put a day's ration of drugs into a small box or container in the morning, so that there is no doubt as to whether a dose has been taken. Special boxes are available which are compartmentalised for this purpose.

The drugs employed in the treatment of epilepsy are not habit-forming, and do not produce a desire to increase the dose. Unfortunately, they are not free from side-effects, which vary in degree and from one individual to another. For example, prolonged administration of the commonly used drug, Phenytoin, can cause swelling of the gums and may affect the development of the teeth in children. This drug, and others, can also cause drowsiness, unsteadiness and lack of co-ordination when a certain concentration in the blood is exceeded. The dose which will produce this varies somewhat from one individual to another. It is now possible to estimate the level of most commonly used anticonvulsant drugs in a sample of blood. By this means toxic reactions can usually be avoided. It is also possible to check that an adequate dose is being given. Sensitivity to drugs is often shown by the development of a skin rash. Other reactions may affect the digestion or bowels.

Children and adolescents may react to drugs in a different way from adults. For instance Phenobarbitone may be calming to an adult, but will cause some children to be very over-active and irritable – a difficulty that has to be taken into consideration when prescribing.

Drugs in combination

Drugs may be used singly or in combination. The effect of combining two drugs is not always simply additive, for one drug sometimes enhances or retards the action of another. For this reason, also, one should be cautious about mixing anti-epileptic medicines with substances taken for other complaints; this includes alcohol, the effect of which may be made much more powerful by some commonly used anticonvulsants. It is essential to tell any doctor, who may be consulted for some other reason, if anti-epileptic medication is being taken if he does not already know. Antibiotics may affect drug activity, and certain combinations can be harmful.

A critical change in the concentration of a substance in the blood may be brought about by the introduction of another anticonvulsant drug (e.g. potentiation of the effect of Phenytoin by Sulthiame, which increases the rate of absorption; other drugs increase the rate of destruction). The effect of adding another anticonvulsant may even be to cause fits to increase in degree and frequency, or to cause toxic reactions. It is therefore most important that drug combinations and dosages should be altered only on medical advice.

Unfortunately, the amount of drugs, or of a single drug, necessary to bring about complete control of fits may be so high that side-effects occur. A compromise has then to be worked out. A minor degree of sedation may be tolerated in some occupations but not in others; it may be responsible for reducing the learning ability and powers of concentration in children, and these factors must be taken into consideration. To a certain extent it is necessary to use trial and error in order to find the drug or combination of drugs which is most suitable for the treatment of a particular person. Some anticonvulsants may make the patient feel drowsy or unsteady on his feet when they are first taken, but as tolerance is acquired these effects diminish or disappear unless he is especially sensitive, in which case the prescription will probably be changed. Strangely, it does not follow that the effectiveness of the drug in controlling attacks is diminished along with the acquisition of tolerance.

Drugs should be looked on as a kind of insurance policy, like cleaning one's teeth. Even when fits have ceased, drugs are usually prescribed for several more years before gradually withdrawing them (under medical supervision). It may not be appreciated by the patient or his relatives that attacks are being prevented or suppressed by the medication, and the thought 'Why am I taking these pills when I no longer have attacks?' may be followed by a demoralising experience if they are stopped and a fit occurs.

The drugs which are used are generally available as liquids for children and in the form of tablets or capsules for adults. There is a large variety, and unfortunately they are marketed under different names by various firms, the name of a particular product not necessarily being the same from country to country.

Before anyone with epilepsy travels abroad he should be sure that he has a good supply of his tablets and that he knows what they are called in the place he is visiting, in case they have to be renewed. If this seems at all likely he should check that his own drugs are available where he is going. This may be done through the International Bureau for Epilepsy (see Appendix, p. 99). A patient should always carry his tablets with him, since after an attack it may be advisable to take an additional dose. Some drugs may have to be given by injection in case of emergency.

Drugs commonly used to treat epilepsy

Phenobarbitone used to be the first choice, although it is now preferred as a stand-by in case of failure with other drugs. It is reliable and cheap, but does have sedative properties and is less well tolerated by children. Names under which it is marketed include Luminal and Gardenal (Garoin also contains Phenytoin).

Phenytoin is the drug of first choice for most prescribers and is closely related to Carbamazepine (Tegretol). Its rate of absorption by the body is variable, and correct dose adjustment is important. Some side-effects of its use have been mentioned. Its rate of metabolisation is slowed by *Sulthiame* (Ospolot), with resulting increased effect. (The metabolisation of phenobarbitone and primidone is also retarded.) Phenytoin is marketed as Epanutin, Dilantin, or Hydantine, among other names.

Primidone (Mysoline) is converted into phenobarbitone in the body, and has proved a useful drug of second choice, with some of the disadvantages of phenobarbitone in consequence of the changes that take place after absorption.

Sodium Valproate (Epilim) is another drug which may be given after Phenytoin has been tried. Unfortunately it is new and therefore expensive, but it may be very useful, especially in children. Its value is still being determined.

Carbamazepine (Tegretol) is chemically similar to Phenytoin but exerts an independent action. It is not usually a first choice of drug, and it is not always beneficial. It may have a dramatic effect on the fit frequency of some patients with major seizures or temporal lobe attacks.

These are the main drugs employed in the treatment of epilepsy. Many other substances are available and may be needed from time to time, but the ones referred to above are those most likely to be used. When serial seizures or status epilepticus occurs, various other substances may be given by injection into the body or infusion into the blood. One need not be concerned with their names here, except to mention Diazepam (Valium) and Chlormethiazole (Heminevrin).

The drugs referred to so far are used for nearly all forms of epilepsy, but true petit-mal responds to the anticonvulsant *Ethosuximide* (Zarontin or Emeside). Sodium Bromide was used in the past, but is no longer prescribed because of its unwanted side-effects and relative inefficiency compared with more recent drugs. The list of drugs and the trade names mentioned are by no means complete, but they are given as a useful sample.

Treatment by surgery

Surgery can remove the cause of epilepsy only if there is a small area of abnormal brain which can be cut away without causing damage or affecting performance. For removal to be a practical proposition, there must be only one such area. Such sources of epilepsy are found most often in the temporal lobes, where they give rise to fits of the same name (*temporal lobe fits*, p. 28). The scars which follow brain injury can sometimes be excised, but although temporary relief may be obtained, the results are often disappointing in the long term. Tumours which give rise to epilepsy can often be removed completely, but, even where the tumour has been taken away, damage to neighbouring cells may be such that a tendency to epilepsy continues, though fits may be prevented by taking tablets. Even more rarely, large areas of brain can be removed if they can be shown to be virtually functionless and also causing fits, or that they impair the normal working of the rest of the brain.

Studies are now being carried out to determine whether epilepsy can be prevented by destroying minute areas of the brain which are responsible for the propagation of the electro-chemical impulses that give rise to an attack. Most of this work has yet to be fully evaluated, but there are signs that effective treatment may be possible for some patients whose fits are resistant to drugs. It is possible to do this kind of (stereotactic) surgery through a small hole in the skull using apparatus which carries an instrument to the spot required without having to open the head widely in order to reach the brain. The electrical activity of deep structures can be recorded at the same time.

Another technique which is still being explored is to stimulate the cerebellum (which is the part of the brain lying in the lowest compartment of the head at the back) by means of electrical impulses generated in an apparatus connected to the surface of that part of the brain. Radio transmission from the surface of the body to a receiver beneath the skin produces currents without the need for wires to pass through the skin itself, thereby avoiding the risk of infection. The impulses generated in the cerebellum by electrical stimulation from outside pass through normal channels within the brain to influence the abnormal activity in those cells which are responsible for producing the patient's fits. So far it appears that very limited benefit is produced by this method.

Other research techniques which may hold promise include methods whereby abnormal electrical activity in the brain can be detected by special sensors which counter the activity by feeding other impulses into the brain. At present this is still in the experimental stage, and it will be years before any technique of this nature can be generally applied, if it proves to be successful.

Research into other alternatives to drug treatment or surgery, such as psychological conditioning, is going on. Acupuncture and similar techniques are tried from time to time. However, no satisfactory substitute for medicines or surgery has yet been found.

Clearly, patients with epilepsy are as liable as other people to depression or any other disturbance of equanimity, which may aggravate the seizures or increase their frequency. Helping to treat these emotional aspects by any other means, whether it be by psychotherapy, faith healing, meditation or anything else, will be of benefit to the patient, and may indeed improve his epilepsy.

Prevention of epilepsy

Better than the development of a more effective means of treating epilepsy would be the discovery of a reliable way of preventing it altogether. Improvement in obstetric technique would reduce the incidence of damage to the child at birth. Better control of infectious diseases and their prevention by inoculation would reduce the likelihood of complications in the brain which may produce fits. Unfortunately, these inoculations are occasionally a cause of brain damage, but apart from whooping-cough and measles vaccines, which should seldom be given to patients who have an abnormal brain for any reason, the risks of damage being produced by the vaccine or inoculation are much less than the risks which are associated with the diseases themselves.

Head injury is one of the most frequent causes of epilepsy, and in the enormous number of road traffic accidents that occur (in seventy per cent of which there are head injuries) we have a demonstrable cause of epilepsy which could be considerably reduced, if not prevented. Protective helmets for motor cyclists effectively reduce the amount of damage which occurs to the head in an accident, although they do not safeguard it completely from injury. The same applies to the use of seat belts in cars. There is a need for very careful design throughout the car, in order to reduce the risks of injury to a minimum.

The size of the problem

Approximately five per cent, or one person in twenty, of the population in the United Kingdom will have an epileptic fit at some time in his life, and there are about three thousand new sufferers each year – some of whom may only have one or two fits and then be free for the rest of their lives. One per cent of all the work days lost through illness is due to epilepsy, while there are twenty-two thousand people, most of whom are under the age of sixty-five, who are in various institutions under continuous medical surveillance, or in special schools in the United Kingdom. The size of the problem is therefore considerable. The people with epilepsy would fill a city the size of Oxford, England, or Charlotte, North Carolina, USA.

CHAPTER SIX

Epilepsy and the Family

There are, as we have seen, so many different ways in which epilepsy can occur and so many different causes of epilepsy, as well as different factors which precipitate an epileptic seizure, that it is unusual to meet two people who have precisely the same experience of the condition. We have already underlined the fact that epilepsy is not a disease in itself and that the epileptic fit is the outward sign of some disordered activity in the brain. For all these reasons it is not practical to talk about 'a typical case' of epilepsy or a 'typical child' with epilepsy, and we have to eschew generalisations wherever we can.

Nevertheless, in almost all cases the announcement that a child has epilepsy is regarded as a calamity. In Oxford a consultant in children's disorders and a social worker studied eighty-one children whose major or only disorder was epilepsy. All except four of the parents concerned expressed fear of the condition or horror on seeing their child for the first time in an epileptic attack. This fear was not limited to people who had had no previous knowledge or experience of epilepsy. Twenty-one of the parents (mainly nurses) had seen an attack previously, but this experience made little difference to their feelings when seeing their own child in this state. In another study by a community physician, this time of infantile convulsions, which are often less dramatic and frightening than major epileptic attacks, it was reported that the first thought of between one-third and one-half of the mothers was that the child was dead or dying.

Another fear is of the diagnosis itself. Owing to inadequate information people suffer from much anxiety about what it means. Two-thirds of the parents in the Oxford study connected epilepsy with some degree of subnormality or insanity. Many children's doctors will have had experience of distraught parents doubting their ability to care for a child with epilepsy. In extreme cases they may reject the child altogether. Much time has to be spent in counselling parents who feel this way and in reassuring them of their ability to cope with their child's disability. It is a common experience that, following swiftly on the shock of hearing the diagnosis, parents begin to seek for a cause. One-quarter of the parents in the Oxford study expressed fears about hereditary aspects. Their own parents and relatives can sometimes aggravate this anxiety and there may be a great deal of anxious examination of the family tree. The routine question in the clinical examination – 'Has any other member of the family had fits?' – lends weight to these fears.

Once again we have to remind ourselves that epilepsy is not one simple condition. Many people who have epilepsy have no record of any sort of fits in any other member of the family. Some types of epilepsy seem to have a slightly higher risk of inheritance. If one parent has epilepsy the risk that the child may have epilepsy varies between 2.5 and 6 per cent. The chances that relatives of a patient may have epilepsy themselves vary between 1.5 and 3 per cent. There are particular circumstances, such as when immunisation is being considered, when it is important to know if epilepsy 'is in the family', but there are far too many occasions when excessive stress is laid on the family history.

Every family is a group of people with varying interests, aims and ambitions. It is not possible for anything which affects one member not to have some greater or lesser influence on the total pattern of activity of the family group. The impact of small events may be less than that of a long-term situation. A condition such as epilepsy, which may well be life-long and carry all sorts of emotional overtones, makes an indelible mark on the family history. When, for example, one of the children has a relatively benign infectious illness there are immediate and short-term alterations in the family's activities. Friends are discouraged from visiting the home, school attendance is halted, plans for excursions and holidays may be interrupted. Such changes may occur when epilepsy is diagnosed and it may be quite a time before the family can completely adapt to this set of circumstances, with which they may have to live for many years. For example, the family may have their choice of holidays limited because a child has epileptic attacks – perhaps they may feel they must travel by car and not for too long distances, or perhaps staying in a guesthouse is too embarrassing following an earlier unhappy experience when a landlady or other guests complained. The occasions when a holiday should have begun with reserved places on a train or other means of transport and had to be postponed at the last moment because of an epileptic attack will generate all sorts of conflicting emotions in the family – possibly hostility towards the 'offender' and guilt on the part of the child who has been the cause of the disruption and disappointment.

Some parents spend a great deal of time worrying about their personal responsibility for this misfortune, this 'blemish' in the family. It is not difficult to understand this anxiety. Nearly one-fifth of the Oxfordshire parents interviewed in the study referred to above feared that the child's fits were caused by some failure on their part during pregnancy or early infancy. Small events become magnified out of all proportion to their significance. There are times when these difficulties become so acute that the marriage may not be able to stand the strain. Recriminations may become so unbearable that a normal relationship cannot continue. Sometimes the father may seek comfort elsewhere if he feels that the child with epilepsy monopolises the mother's attention, to his own exclusion. Such emotions in the parents lead to extremes of behaviour towards the child with epilepsy. The natural desire to protect one's child from harm when faced with epilepsy, a situation of potential danger to the child at any time and in any place, can drive a parent to being over-anxious about his safety.

This is not wholly unreasonable and those concerned in trying to help the family have to be careful that they do not, without proper thought, label the parents as over-protective and so add another dimension to their difficulties. Nevertheless, this natural anxiety has repercussions on other members of the family. Any suggestion that the child with epilepsy receives especially favoured treatment, that he is not expected to do things which siblings have to do, or that he is allowed to get away with misbehaviour because his mother is afraid he might have an epileptic attack if denied what he wants to do, creates difficulties between him and his brothers or sisters. All these emotions will affect family life and will have their influence on the child's development.

Alternatively, he may find it difficult to accept it if his younger siblings do better at school than he does, or surpass him in any other way. This may also lead to friction in the home. Another difficulty arises when siblings go out of the home with friends and do not include him in their games and activities. It can also happen that their friends may not wish to come into the home or may be discouraged by their own parents from doing so.

There have been a number of attempts to measure attitudes towards children and adults with epilepsy. The most reliable recent study was conducted by the Gallup organisation in the United Kingdom in March 1979. Two questions were asked:

'Would you object to having any of your children associate in school or elsewhere with people who sometimes had seizures [fits] or not?'

'Do you think people with epilepsy should or should not be employed in jobs like other people?'

A similar enquiry with almost identical wording was carried out in November 1969. A comparison of the two results gives rise to some hope that efforts to improve the general understanding of epilepsy do produce positive results. At the same time one also hopes that there will be no relaxing in these efforts more especially as the latest poll showed a greater degree of adverse attitudes in the sixteen to twenty-four years age group. The answer to the questions were as follows:

First question:

	Would object	Would not object	Don't know
1969	15 %	68 %	17 %
1979	5 %	88 %	7 %

Second question:

	Should be employed	Should not	Don't know
1969	57 %	23 %	20 %
1979	78 %	12 %	10 %

In Chapter 4 we discussed the concept of 'epileptic personality', which was quite popular for some time, but is now fairly generally discarded. It was suggested by the proponents of this concept that having epilepsy meant that the patient also had many disagreeable characteristics and that it was better to avoid his company. Children are not likely to advance this as a reason for avoiding another child who is subject to attacks but, as can be seen, this sort of thinking has led parents to be anxious about exposing their children to the companionship of a child suffering from epilepsy. Similarly, while some adults may be genuinely concerned about the risk to someone with epilepsy working in certain industries there are undoubtedly some people who cannot tolerate the thought of working alongside an 'epileptic'. The complex and varied factors in the constitution of any individual with epilepsy make it questionable whether there is ever any justification in calling someone an 'epileptic'. In Chapter 3 we discussed some causes of the condition and we showed that in some people a cause can be found. It seems probable that many people have a predisposition towards epileptic fits, but if they are fortunate the appropriate provocation, be it illness, a head injury or part of the process of ageing, will not occur, and they will avoid epileptic attacks. The idea that all men are born equal but some are more equal than others might be paraphrased to 'All are born epileptic but some are more epileptic than others'.

We said earlier that a mother usually learns fairly soon how to look after her child with epilepsy. The stresses and strains on family life vary tremendously. While one can never ignore the risk that once a child has had an epileptic attack he might have another, there is a constantly increasing possibility that attacks can be controlled and sometimes it is possible to be fairly confident that they will not recur. Many small children have one odd convulsion. Epilepsy is not diagnosed from one attack. But even where the diagnosis is confirmed by further attacks it is not the end of the world, it is not a sentence for life, which many parents thought it was in the past. Given adequate medical and social guidance most families can cope and do cope very well indeed.

CHAPTER SEVEN

Epilepsy in School and After

For many parents of children with epilepsy the time when the child must start going to school is one of very great difficulty. The risk of seizures occurring in many different situations such as when travelling on the school bus, crossing a major road with all the traffic hazards, or even in the school playground, is very small but mothers are understandably anxious in spite of this reassurance. It is usually the mother who has to make the daily decision whether the child should go to school or whether his state of health warrants keeping him at home. Father will have departed for work, possibly after announcing that the child must not be molly-coddled. It is not difficult to see how anxiety about these questions so readily leads to over-protective attitudes on one side and possibly parental friction. Counselling is very necessary at this stage since parents are frequently subjected to criticism by family, neighbours and authorities both for being too fearful of risks or not sufficiently attentive to them.

Parents are not the only ones to have anxious moments. Teachers frequently question the extent of their responsibility if a child has a seizure in the classroom, in the gymnasium or in some other situation of potential danger, such as being near a hot-plate in the cookery class. They ask if it is safe to include a child with epilepsy on a school journey. At the same time they must have regard to the disappointment and frustration of a child who is left out of school activities to which his companions are admitted. Teachers are often worried

about questions of discipline and punishment for bad behaviour - is punishment likely to provoke an epileptic attack?
However much one may assure the teacher that disciplining a
child is less detrimental to him than allowing him to avoid
the normal consequences of misdeeds and possibly growing
up a maladjusted adolescent, the teacher will still be subject to
conflicting emotions and may feel responsible for causing an
attack to occur.

These are real problems which play a part sometimes
greater, sometimes smaller, in the development of any child
who is subject to seizures either major or minor. It is estimated
that there are between 65,000 and 70,000 children of school
age in Britain who are either having epileptic attacks or
receiving medication to keep these attacks under control.
There is also a small group of children who do not have any
overt form of attack, but whose EEG records demonstrate
considerable disorderly activity in the brain cells and who
may be said to have sub-clinical attacks. These may interfere
with learning at school in the same way as a brief interruption
in a telephone conversation can cause any of us to feel
confused. The child may be classified as inattentive or lazy.
This may also be the case in petit-mal (see p. 28). A substantial
proportion of sufferers from petit-mal are subject to disturbed
behaviour which is thought to be caused by the disorder.

Just under one per cent of the 65-70,000 children quoted
above will be found in the five special residential schools for
children with epilepsy. The largest of these in the United
Kingdom is the Lingfield Hospital School in Surrey where
there are places for 280 children. Lingfield also has an adolescent training unit for forty young people. The remaining
residential schools are as follows:

Coulthurst School (David Lewis Centre) Cheshire	100
Chilton School (Maghull Homes) Lancashire	60
St Elizabeth's School, Herts.	60
Sedgwick House School, Cumbria	40

Plans are in hand for a new residential school in North-East

England, particularly reducing the need for children to travel far from home and alleviating the difficulties of parents in making regular visits to them. Quarriers Homes in Scotland has a residential unit for children with epilepsy. These children attend the special day school maintained in the grounds of the Homes by the local authority.

Broadly speaking, it is thought that 500-600 places meet the needs of those children who require special residential accommodation on medical grounds. It is not so certain that this number is sufficient for those children who require special help on educational grounds. There is particular concern that those children who are multiply handicapped will not do well in non-specialist schools. There is a trend of thought that all children attending special schools should eventually be placed in ordinary schools. This is to be welcomed in so far as it is a move away from segregation of children with any form of disability.

It is not by any means the end of the story to find that the majority of children with epilepsy are attending ordinary schools, although this in itself is a substantial achievement and a situation which is a great deal better than in many other countries. What of course is important is to know how they get on in these schools. A number of people have been trying to find the answer to this question. A study in a Midlands county in England found that half the children were achieving only an indifferent level and that no more than one-third were making satisfactory progress. This means that one child in six was having considerable difficulty in keeping up with school work. This group of children included many with behaviour disorders and other handicaps.

Professor Neville Butler's survey of school children in Bristol (Kenneth Gibson Memorial Lecture reported in *Candle*, Journal of the British Epilepsy Association, autumn 1972) looked at poor school performance. He excluded from his figures children who were severely retarded or brain damaged but even so he found that among children attending normal schools who have already had a fit by the age of seven years, very nearly twice as many do badly on a simple test when compared with children who are not affected. A full and comprehensive study of school children in the Isle of Wight has shown that children with epilepsy are on average twenty months behind their peers.

The reasons for this unsatisfactory state of affairs are many and various. It is believed that anti-epileptic drugs play some part in impeding performance, but the evidence as to how far this is so is not clear. Some children with epilepsy miss time at school not only as the result of parental anxiety, but also because they need a day or two at home after a bad epileptic attack. Frequent hospital attendance can also account for time lost. Children who suffer from minor forms of epileptic attack (or 'absences') may appear to be fully physically capable of being in school, but it is known that such attacks can interfere with concentration and memory retention, and in many subtle ways interfere with school progress. The effect of sub-clinical attacks has been mentioned on p. 58.

Finally, poor achievement may be the outcome of the child being allowed too easy a passage through school. Mention has been made of the anxiety expressed by some teachers that their actions may provoke epileptic attacks. Having heard that stress is undesirable the teacher may interpret this to mean that the child should not be put under any pressure. We will come back to this again. Meanwhile, we should always be careful not to exaggerate the significance of 'stress' in the life of someone with epilepsy. Information for teachers on this and other aspects of the child with epilepsy in school is available from the British Epilepsy Association.

Once again, as so often with this condition, there is no clear and simple answer to the problem of education and epilepsy. It was once a common misconception that a child with seizures was a mentally sub-normal child. Needless to say, if one visits a hospital for the mentally handicapped one will find children who are severely sub-normal and who have epileptic attacks. In fact about 25 per cent of seriously mentally handicapped people will be subject to some type of epileptic fit - and quite often to very severe epilepsy. The initial damage to the brain, possibly the result of birth injury or of a severe illness in the first months of the child's life, is in such cases responsible for both mental handicap and epilepsy. In a small number of tragic cases the child may have cerebral palsy as well.

An examination of children living at home and receiving treatment from the family doctor or hospital out-patient clinic will produce very much the same range of high, average and low intelligence as in the general population of children. There have been outstanding geniuses and national heroes with epilepsy throughout the history of mankind and there is no reason why this should not continue to be so.

Epileptic attacks in school

Wherever possible the child with epilepsy should attend the school he would have entered if he were not subject to epileptic attacks. A child who is properly occupied within the limits of his capacity may well be less subject to epileptic attacks than if he is under-occupied, bored and unhappy. It is clearly important that his teachers be given the fullest information about what sort of attacks he is likely to have, what they may mean to the child and what action the teachers should be prepared to take.

The most common form of epilepsy the school teacher will see is that involving major seizures. Fortunately these respond most readily to anti-epileptic medication so that they do not occur as frequently as they might. Even so, the teacher will want to know what he or she should do.

First aid for epilepsy is discussed on pp. 42-43. If a fit occurs in the classroom it is particularly important that the teacher should remain calm and unflustered. Children become disturbed, anxious and even hostile more readily if they see the adult in their midst is in a panic at the sight of an attack. It is useful to make notes of what actually occurs since such observations may be valuable to the doctor in establishing a diagnosis. Since some parents cannot give a clear and objective account of what happens, the teacher may be the only reliable witness. The teacher may also find that what is a new and surprising experience for him is by no means new in the life of the family. One of the consequences of the misunderstandings, fears and prejudices about epilepsy is that the family may not wish to disclose the fact that their child has epilepsy until there is no possibility of concealing it.

Other forms of epileptic attack do not require so much active intervention from the teacher, but they call for tolerance and acceptance which may be more difficult. For example the child who makes loud noises while smacking his lips in a focal attack can be almost more disturbing than the child who falls on the floor in a convulsion. It may be difficult for the teacher to know whether autonomic behaviour is unconscious or simulated. Other children may provide a mock attack as a diversion to class routine. The control of a class of high-spirited children under such circumstances can be difficult. It is hoped that these problems will not be made the excuse for turning the child away from the school he should be attending.

A small number of children will be subject to the brief absences of consciousness lasting three to five seconds which are true petit-mal. Such children not only miss what is said in these brief absences, but may not be able to remember what was said immediately before the attack. For a child suffering from this type of epilepsy it may be necessary to repeat information, particularly where this includes instructions about future activities. A simple example from the headmaster of one special school is that the child may hear the teacher say 2 and 2 (is 4; 3 and 3) is 6 – that is, he is only aware of what is outside the brackets. He may well be convinced that this is what the teacher said, the resulting difficulties between him and his teacher being added to the cumulative effect of numerous misunderstandings of this nature.

Some thought should be given to what sort of school activities are permitted to the child with epilepsy, and from which activities he should be excluded. Two considerations are important: first, that embargoes should be as few as possible: secondly, that we must constantly remind ourselves that it is seldom that any two children are alike in fit frequency, in type of fits, in what provokes fits, in personality and in capacity to cope with their own condition or accept it. Having shown that generalisations are rarely valid the following points should be considered.

If a child who is currently subject to epileptic attacks wishes to swim, it is desirable to obtain the agreement of the parents and the school doctor before allowing him to do so. It is also important that there should be at least two adults present if the child is in the swimming bath with the rest of the class. It is not reasonable for one adult to supervise a large group and also give special attention to one child who might need urgent help to get out of the bath if he has an attack. Accidents in these circumstances are extremely rare but the emergency is a real one if the child should get into difficulties.

Similarly with physical education: a child subject to epilepsy who is actively engaged on wall bars, ropes and other equipment very rarely comes to any harm under proper supervision. The girl in the domestic science class, the boy in the carpentry class, may be facing some additional risks, but these should not be over-estimated. It is well to be sure once again that parents and the school doctor know what is going on and are in agreement with these activities. Wherever possible the child with epilepsy should follow the same programme as his peers, provided that obvious risks are guarded against as unobtrusively as possible. The more he is singled out for special treatment, the more activities he is excluded from, the more he is likely to have social difficulties in the future.

The main reason why some children with epilepsy are slow is the underlying brain damage which can be responsible for the attacks. In general these children have little difficulty in following an ordinary school programme which is suitable to their mental level. Teachers are sometimes concerned about pressing the child to work harder. The answer lies, as it so often does, in what is a reasonable expectation for a particular child. There is very rarely any harm in urging him to work to his full capacity. In an extreme case, a young person with limited intellectual capacity caught up in his parents' desire for him to pass 'O' level examinations which are clearly beyond him, may have renewed epileptic attacks. In such circumstances it may be necessary to advise him and his parents to aim at more modest targets.

Many a young student without any disability may find examinations, and preparation for them, a time of stress. A young person with epilepsy may become anxious and possibly more vulnerable to attacks, but this is not a good argument for excusing him the normal stressful experience which others have to face. It is desirable to see that the stress is not excessive. Where necessary extra time and other facilities can be arranged with the headmaster and the examining body. Care should be taken that he gets his normal quota of food and rest and is not burning the candle at both ends.

Epilepsy in adolescence

Well before he is due to leave school, the child with epilepsy – and indeed with any disability – should be preparing for a future career. In the experience of many careers officers it is important that the young man or woman should be able to offer some skill to offset what may be considered to be the disqualifying factor of a disability. This is more particularly true where the disability is one which does not readily arouse sympathy, as it does in the case of a blind girl or a partly paralysed young man. It is certainly desirable that a boy or girl with epilepsy should be prepared well ahead of the day he or she leaves the sheltered atmosphere of school.

Before considering employment in more detail it is as well to look at the particular situation of the young adolescent who has epilepsy. Adolescence is for everyone a time of great change. The boy suddenly finds he speaks with a deep voice: worse still there are times when he does not know what sort of noise will come out when he opens his mouth to speak. Boys and girls develop exciting but alarming new physical characteristics. New thoughts arise unbidden and sometimes without warning. The adults with whom one has contact are unpredictable - at times they treat one as a grown-up with responsibilities - at other times they deny that these exist. One may be old enough to be the father of a child but not old enough to get married. If, in the boy's first attempts to get to know the other sex, his girl friend becomes pregnant he is in real trouble, but if he does not mix with girls or like meeting them, he is thought not to be normal. He rebels against authority and wants to eat, drink and dress as he wishes. He does not want to conform to the behaviour which parents expect or do what an old person like the teacher or the doctor tells him to do.

So the chief characteristics of adolescence are change, uncertainty, confusion and rebellion. And epilepsy is a condition in which something dramatic and disturbing may happen at any moment, and often without warning. Epilepsy is also confusing and strewn with conflicting advice. Parents have been advised to let the young person grow up like any other child, and take no special notice of the epilepsy, but at the same time he has to take his tablets, he may not be allowed to lock the bathroom door when taking a bath, and he may not be able to drive a car or a motor-cycle like his friends.

It is not surprising that parents often complain about the impossible behaviour of their adolescent child with epilepsy. How often do all parents experience some difficulty in dealing with their children as they grow through adolescence, without having the additional problem of coping with epilepsy?

At all stages - at home, going to school and during adolescence - the child or young person with epilepsy demands an extra measure of tolerance, patience and good humour if the process of growing up is not to result in an individual who is out of tune with everyone around him, carrying a larger than life-size chip on his shoulder and doomed to difficulties and disappointments wherever he goes.

CHAPTER EIGHT

Employment

We have repeatedly said that epilepsy is not one single condition, nor does it appear in the same form in everyone who has epilepsy. Nevertheless, many people with epilepsy experience difficulty at some time or another in obtaining employment. The British Epilepsy Association Advice Service receives several thousand enquiries each year. Chief among these are questions concerning employment. In their survey of epilepsy in general practices Pond and Bidwell found that 64 out of 157 patients of employable age had *serious* difficulties with employment at some time. A smaller survey of epilepsy in rural areas suggested that difficulties might be less in the country than in the town and that most adults were able to secure some form of employment. Nevertheless it is rare to meet someone who can truly say that having or having had epilepsy has not played some part in his or her working life.

The common attitude of the uninformed employer towards epilepsy is as follows: he appreciates there is a problem in finding the right sort of employment: he really wishes he could help the applicant, but his workshop, office or trade is not geared to taking on someone who has epilepsy. He may be concerned about the amount of risk involved, whether it will affect his insurance policy, whether the members of his staff will accept 'an epileptic' as a colleague at work, whether such a person can be relied on in times of special difficulties and a number of other factors. Sometimes the employer may be right, but more often his anxiety about the consequences of epilepsy in the workplace is unjustified and it is possible to give him evidence that this is so.

More difficult to deal with, and even less justified, is the employer who says he would like to help the applicant, but that previous experience of employing 'an epileptic' has convinced him that there is no room for such people in his employ. We have stressed that a typical case of epilepsy does not exist but this is still far from being appreciated. An employer who has had an earlier unfortunate experience with someone who was mentally handicapped as well as having epilepsy may lay the blame on the wrong condition. An illustration of this was the employer, a jam manufacturer, who had employed a young mentally handicapped woman to sweep up the floors in his factory. This girl was also 'a known epileptic'. One day, during a row with the supervisor about sweeping up a broken bottle, she tossed the contents of her dustpan over her shoulder and into a vat of preserves. It is doubtful whether epilepsy had anything to do with the incident, but the employer was not to be moved from his determination that he would never employ another 'epileptic'. On the other hand, where an employer has had a conscientious, hard worker whose epileptic attacks are reasonably well controlled he is frequently willing to give someone else a chance.

The selection of suitable employment reaches back into the years at school and forward into adult life. It is imperative that the reasons for any decision about the suitability or otherwise of employment for an individual with epilepsy should be sound and valid. Too often they are not.

There is a notable tendency to recommend 'easy' or 'safe' occupations for the young person who has epilepsy. Sometimes this can be carried to absurd lengths. In a recent case before an industrial tribunal the local authority argued that it was unsafe for a young librarian to work in a library because it was necessary to climb steps when returning books to the top shelves. It was pointed out that in most modern libraries books are contained in shelves which can be reached by the librarian and the user of the library without the use of steps or if need be with very small steps as opposed to long ladders.

The range is wide and it is more practical to instance those jobs which are unsuitable. A study of patients attending a hospital neurology clinic (which meant that they were subject to frequent attacks or to more severe and complex types of epilepsy) showed that 164 patients held a hundred different types of occupation. Another study at a large motor company found 55 men with epilepsy among the 21,075 employed. Their job classifications were as follows:

Production	12
Supply	4
Labouring	7
Machinists	6
Staff	5
Bench Work	5
Stores	3
Tool-room fitters	2
Inspectors	2
Miscellaneous	9

Dr Ivan MacIntyre undertook a survey in conjunction with the British Epilepsy Association and the North-West Group of the Society of Occupational Medicine and collected information from twenty-nine works doctors regarding about 150,000 people at work. 177 employees were known to have epilepsy. The twenty-nine companies varied from heavy engineering, coal, gas and steel production to food and chemicals.

An ABC of employment and epilepsy might be constructed as follows:

AIRMAN   *No* if one has epilepsy or has ever had epilepsy.

ARCHITECT   *Yes* if one has epilepsy but *no* if one has not obtained three 'A' Levels.

BARMAN
Yes. No problem if epilepsy is reasonably well controlled.

BIOLOGIST
Yes. No problem with epilepsy providing one has the ability to pass the appropriate examinations.

BUILDING WORKER
Yes. No problem but preferably epilepsy controlled for three years if it involves work on scaffolding. May need a driving licence to get to work so again will need three years freedom from attacks.

BUS DRIVER
No if one has had an attack since the age of three years.

CHARTERED ACCOUNTANT
Yes if educational qualifications are appropriate.

CIVIL SERVICE
Yes. There is no absolute bar to someone with a history of epilepsy being accepted for a post in the Civil Service. Consideration is given to the type of post which is being applied for in relation to the type of epilepsy, period of freedom from attacks, etc.

CLERGYMAN
Yes. Personality and intellectual level are more important than epilepsy – but again mobility and ability to hold a driving licence may be significant.

DOCK WORKER
Yes, but must be well-controlled for at least three years. An early history of epilepsy is not relevant.

ENGINE DRIVER
No if one has epilepsy or has ever had epilepsy.

FARM WORKER
Yes. It may be necessary to hold a driving licence but otherwise no problems.

GARDENER
Yes.

HEAVY GOODS VEHICLE DRIVER
No if applicant has had any attacks after the age of three years.

LECTURER
Yes. Epilepsy rarely relevant.

LIBRARIAN
Yes. In connection with the appearance

before an Industrial Tribunal referred to previously, the British Epilepsy Association obtained information from 177 libraries and found that forty libraries had between them fifty people with epilepsy in their employment. (Thirty-five were public libraries and five were university libraries.) Well over half of those employed were library assistants and nine were qualified librarians. The only reported instance of an applicant being refused was someone who could not drive a motor vehicle because of continuing epileptic attacks.

MERCHANT NAVY *No.*

MIDWIFE The Central Midwives Board have recently agreed that an applicant for registration as a certified midwife must have been free from epileptic attacks for two years without taking medication. This last qualification in acceptance is under discussion.

NURSE *Yes.* There are many nurses who are successful in spite of a history of epilepsy. It is not possible to list exact requirements in regard to health and educational level as this varies from hospital to hospital. In the main acceptance for training depends on the judgement of the Director of the School of Nursing and a favourable report from a specialist.

OCCUPATIONAL THERAPIST *Yes.* Epilepsy is not recognised as a disqualification. Personality and educational level (requiring two 'A' levels, usually in English and Biology) are more relevant.

PHARMACIST   *Yes.* There is no reason why someone with a history of epilepsy which is reasonably well-controlled should not train as a pharmacist. Here again it is necessary for any applicant to have passed three 'A' levels which should include either Chemistry, Biology, Zoology or Physics and this is more relevant than the epilepsy.

SOLDIER   The armed forces now consider applicants with a history of epilepsy if the applicant has been free from attacks for several years and depending on which branch the applicant wishes to join.

TEACHER   *Yes.* The Department of Education and Science circular 4/75 says that a person who has been subject to epilepsy should not for this reason alone be excluded from training as a teacher if he has been free from fits for a period of approximately three years. Students or, or qualified teachers in, physical education may be required to have a longer period of freedom from fits. Posts in private education are at the discretion of governing bodies or head teachers.

We could continue the list to include secretaries, social workers, shop assistants, solicitors, warehousemen and weavers. It is simpler to describe *unsuitable* employment. Certain jobs where there is a potential hazard may have to be regarded as undesirable for some people but possibly not for everyone with a history of epilepsy. As we have indicated above, a great deal will depend on the type of epilepsy, the frequency of attacks, the time of their occurrence, the form they take, whether the sufferer knows when an attack is about to take place and the sort of person he is.

For someone who has frequent attacks occurring without

warning one could not recommend work near dangerous and unguarded heavy machinery nor work at heights or over water (e.g. at the dockside) or in control of moving vehicles. Having said this, one has to admit that even in these types of employment there are exceptions, as for example one patient who was an experienced steeplejack with an accident-free record for more than twenty years. Clearly, however, we would not advise a young person with epilepsy to take up this occupation nor would a careers officer take the responsibility for doing so. Regard must also be paid to the safety of others which might be imperilled by someone having an attack, for example, while working on scaffolding. Tragic accidents where someone below has been permanently or fatally injured by a tool or equipment being dropped by a worker who has not got epilepsy cause the employer to hesitate to employ at heights someone who is known to have epilepsy. Recent legislation regarding health and safety at work require the employer to give proper consideration to this.

The information collected by Dr Ivan MacIntyre referred to previously provides some figures about frequency of accidents. He reports that only eighteen accidents were attributed to epilepsy in the twenty-nine factories over approximately ten years. The accident frequency rate is defined as lost time in accidents multiplied by 100,000 and divided by the man hours worked. In this case the accident frequency rate of the workers who had epilepsy was 0.06. Dr MacIntyre acknowledges that there are pitfalls when comparing accident statistics of different companies, but draws attention to figures from the British Chemicals Industry (1972) where twenty-nine companies employing over 1,000 people each reported an accident frequency rate between 0.09 and 4.64 with an average of 1.92. He comments: 'One cannot conclude that the way to reduce accidents is to employ only people with epilepsy, but certainly it is abundantly clear that those with epilepsy in this survey do not play any significant part in accident causation.' ('Epilepsy and employment', in *Community Health*, Journal of The Royal Institute of Public Health and Hygiene, Vol. 7, No. 4, April 1976.)

Advice and aid in finding employment are available to everyone who is disabled from all Employment Offices and Job Centres of the Employment Service Agency, including anyone with epilepsy – either as his or her principal disability or when epilepsy is associated with other health problems. The Employment Service Agency maintains a register which contains the names of people regarded as substantially handicapped in obtaining employment. Registration is entirely voluntary and every individual applicant is completely free to make his own attempts to find employment. Many people with well-controlled epilepsy do obtain employment without registering. The Disabled Persons (Employment) Act 1944, requires employers of twenty or more people to have a percentage of registered disabled persons, so that someone who is substantially handicapped is well advised to register and obtain the help of the Disablement Resettlement Officer (DRO). The services of the DRO are, in fact, available to all disabled people and not only to those on the register.

The Agency has published a leaflet, *Employing Someone with Epilepsy,* which is available to all employers. It gives information about the person with epilepsy in the workplace and gives practical guidance in dealing with such problems as may arise. The DRO is available for consultation by any employer wishing to employ a disabled person and is frequently well-informed on the problems associated with epilepsy, since a regular feature of his training is the provision of information about this condition. Where it is felt to be in the interest of the applicant who has epilepsy, he can be referred for a course of industrial rehabilitation. For those with the appropriate capacity a course can be offered in a Skills Centre or in one of four residential training colleges, or in a number of technical and commercial colleges and colleges of further education.

The training opportunities for young disabled people improve year by year and anyone with epilepsy is strongly recommended to consult the Careers Officer or the Disablement Resettlement Officer about these. The Advice Service at the British Epilepsy Association can offer further information in this area.

In recent years the DRO has had the benefit of the Employment Medical Advisory Service (EMAS) which is part of the Health and Safety Executive of the Department of Employment. EMAS is at present making a careful study of the impact of a number of different disorders on employment, and high on their list of such disorders is epilepsy. A survey of the factors affecting successful placement after training or re-training has been carried out and guidelines regarding the employment of people with epilepsy are in course of preparation.

The employer who takes on someone with epilepsy on the recommendation of the DRO can be confident that the applicant is reasonably well prepared for employment and has every likelihood of being well motivated to make the best of the job offered him. The DRO does not recommend an applicant without first securing his agreement to the disclosure of the nature of his disability to the prospective employer, so removing another of the anxieties of most employers about foreknowledge of what to expect. Most employers have expressed satisfaction at the work performance of the properly selected and placed man or woman with a history of epilepsy. In the majority of cases previous difficulties in securing employment mean that the individual is less likely to give in to stray whims and fancies and more likely to persevere at his work unless he encounters major difficulties.

In a number of organisations the works medical officer has found it beneficial to prepare those working in immediate contact with the new recruit with a few simple facts about his epilepsy – always with his consent. The unexpectedness of an epileptic attack is a potent factor in disruption of work and the creation of all sorts of difficulties. Some medical officers ask an experienced and older employee to act as 'uncle' to the new recruit, especially if he is in his first employment, and to make it clear that no one else need be involved if he should have an attack at work.

It cannot be gainsaid that some people with epilepsy are not good employees, just as some workers who do not have epilepsy do not give satisfaction. Among the (fortunately small) group of people with epilepsy who have a poor work record will be found several who have multiple handicaps. In a study of a hundred people with epilepsy on the Disabled Persons Register who had not secured employment over a period of three months or more in spite of the DRO's strenuous efforts, the late Dr Robert Porter (Central Middlesex Hospital) found that thirty-seven were not likely to obtain employment because of personality or behaviour disorders, low intelligence or other physical disability, and that epilepsy played only a small part in their difficulties. Strangely enough, he found that five had not got epilepsy at all, and that one of these obtained employment the day after he had been freed from the label!

In case one should think that frequency of epileptic attacks is the governing factor in obtaining employment, it is interesting to note that Dr Ernst Rodin (Michigan, USA) studying employment prognosis for the Vocational Rehabilitation Service in that state, found that eighty-eight patients with epilepsy were employed and eighty-four were unemployed. He analysed these to find that of those with less than one fit a year, thirty-two were employed and twelve were unemployed, as one might expect. He also found, however, that of those with several fits a week thirteen were employed and nineteen unemployed: all of which lends strength to the view that in most cases it is not the epilepsy which creates the employment difficulties, although it undoubtedly exacerbates them.

Certainly epilepsy is bedevilled by many myths at all stages. The fear that it might be inherited led to laws forbidding the marriage of people with epilepsy. In underdeveloped countries the fear that epilepsy is infectious leads to the complete social isolation of the epileptic child from the rest of the family. In our culture our fears and taboos may be less dramatic, but various myths are at the foundation of attitudes towards people with epilepsy.

For a very long time it has been stated and believed that people with epilepsy should not work near machinery. This has led some firms to refuse opportunities to people with epilepsy when the machine has been small and of little obvious danger. The law requires adequate guards on industrial machinery and these, in many cases, would be sufficient to prevent someone harming himself in an epileptic attack. Very little has been done to ascertain which way someone falls in an epileptic attack, but a simple count of residents in a centre for people with severe epilepsy showed that more than one half fell backwards, another group fell sideways and backwards and only a small number fell forward. This is an area in which social research might usefully be pursued.

There is a great shortage of accurate information about the social effects on people with epilepsy. The study carried out by Dr MacIntyre has marked a very useful step forward but, as he admits, leaves many questions unanswered. One of the main difficulties of social research is that the object of one's study can never be fitted into a test-tube or on to a slide for detailed inspection. It is possibly for this reason that there have been many more studies which are more medically than socially orientated. The British Epilepsy Association and the Department of Health are jointly supporting a study of the progress of the school leaver who has epilepsy, particularly in regard to his success in obtaining the right sort of employment.

The view has been expressed in the past that people with epilepsy should not be subject to strain because it might precipitate further fits. Recent research is beginning to show that concentration on certain tasks may produce activity in the brain cells which in turn may *reduce* fits. It has been known for a long time that people who are bored, frustrated and depressed by social difficulties become prone to more fits: the phrase that has been coined that 'the best treatment for epilepsy is work' bears considerable truth, as indeed it does for a number of conditions. There is little evidence that people with epilepsy are not able to carry out managerial responsibilities but there are still people who think that promotion to higher responsibility is harmful for someone with epilepsy.

There are anecdotes in support of the view that someone with epilepsy may have an increase of fit frequency when taking up a new appointment. There is need for a controlled study to ascertain whether this is so. It may well be that all the other factors concerned with adolescence and leaving school may combine to make epileptic attacks more frequent at this time, and that going to work has little to do with the attacks.

To sum up, it seems that most people with epilepsy can take part in most forms of work for which their intelligence, aptitude and personality qualify them. Variations in achievement may be in part due to variations in type of epilepsy, but are more often due to the other factors already referred to. There is no doubt that the majority of people with epilepsy are fully able-bodied between attacks, and that, given the opportunity, they may be able to help other handicapped people in the workplace.

In very many cases the time lost as a result of epilepsy is less than the time lost after a family celebration or an evening out with colleagues from the office. Many people with epilepsy value their freedom from attacks too highly to take risks mixing alcohol with their medication or indulging in many late-night parties. They are therefore less likely to suffer from the consequences of over-indulgence and more likely to be good time-keepers and regular at work, and this compensates for the occasional time off necessitated by an epileptic attack.

CHAPTER NINE

Epilepsy and Life

In the previous chapter we touched on some aspects of living with epilepsy. Many people with epilepsy appear to accept their situation with little fuss or bother and very often their casual acquaintances would not think themselves in the company of 'an epileptic' whatever that may mean to them. One does not wish to do or say anything to undermine the self-confidence of people with epilepsy and their adjustment to the problems of living with epilepsy. However, it is difficult to believe that the uncertainties of epilepsy, the unpredictability of epileptic attacks, the disturbance which these have meant in the past and may still mean in the future - that all these have no influence on the individual's attiiude to himself or to life in the community.

Most young people with epilepsy, in common with their peers, want to be accepted in their particular group, but to be an individual, different in clothes, appearance and so on. They want to choose their own area of being different and not to have this forced on them by something over which they have no control. Benny Jacobsen, the Danish architect, describes how, when he could not go on to high school because of ill-health, his friends brought him the traditional high school cap worn by Danish students. They had sensed that the deprivation of this status symbol was a great hardship to him. Similarly, many young people look forward to the day when, like their friends, they can ride a motor cycle or drive a car. There is a great sense of status in being able to take one's girl friend out in a car. Limitations on the possibility of doing so can be a source of frustration and unhappiness, which in turn affects all other relationships.

The law relating to driving licences is under constant review. This is fortunate because for many years, although the appropriate act stated that anyone 'suffering from epilepsy' should not be granted a driving licence, there was much confusion about what 'suffering from epilepsy' actually meant. At one time it was possible to obtain a licence in one county and to be refused a licence in the next county or county borough. There was much scope for the prejudices of the people concerned in making decisions. Some medical officers of health seemed to think that their role was to protect the aged pedestrian, your elderly relative and mine, against the selfishness of epileptics driving juggernauts on our highways. Then, following the ruling of Lord Chief Justice, came a period during which people taking anti-epileptic drugs were *ipso facto* considered to be suffering from epilepsy. This encouraged people with epilepsy to stop taking medication (thus rendering themselves more likely to have seizures) in order to obtain a driving licence.

The present regulations in Britain, introduced in 1970 and since modified, provide that a driving licence may be granted to an applicant who has suffered from or is suffering from epilepsy if he can satisfy the following conditions:

(a) He shall have been free from any epileptic attack whilst awake for at least three years from the date when the licence is to have effect.

(b) In the case of an applicant who has had such attacks while asleep during that period, he shall have been subject to such attacks whilst asleep, but not whilst awake since before the beginning of that period.

(c) The driving of a vehicle by him in pursuance of the licence is not likely to be a source of danger to the public.

In considering the period of freedom from attack, the law in Britain and some other countries no longer requires the applicant to have ceased taking drugs. If the above conditions are fulfilled he may apply, whether he is taking tablets or not. However, should the medication be changed, or reduced, driving should be discontinued for six to twelve months, until evidence of freedom from attacks is again established. If a fit should occur either during the time of changing medication or at any other time the initial rule applies again and three years freedom from attacks is required unless there are very exceptional reasons.

Those people who are on medication should be very careful of the effects of drug interaction, particularly the enhancement of their drugs by alcohol. The best course of action is to avoid alcohol altogether, especially before driving even for a short distance. The need for people on medication to continue to take their drugs regularly without missing a single dose is obvious.

Regulations regarding the issue of licences for the driving of public service vehicles and heavy goods vehicles state that an applicant may not be granted such a licence if he has any epileptic attack after the age of three years. Although the regulations do not cover taxi drivers, many of the local authorities who issue hackney carriage licences apply the same rule.

However, for all general purposes fits before the age of three can be ignored, as can an attack related to illness in childhood from which there has been complete recovery. If there has been any sort of an attack during adolescence it is wise to seek medical advice before applying for a licence.

These new regulations are a great deal more satisfactory. Reviews going on at present may make them even more acceptable to everyone concerned. Plainly there must be some control over licences so issued, but it is imperative that controls are based on scientific evidence of the need for them and not on prejudice on the part of individuals.

If a licence has been granted to someone with a history of epilepsy, it is important to avoid any circumstance, such as hunger or tiredness, which may make the occurrence of an attack more likely.

Even when they have obtained a driving licence some people experience difficulty obtaining the insurance cover they require. There are a number of insurance brokers who specialise in insurance for disabled people, including people with a history of epilepsy. Information about these can be obtained from the British Epilepsy Association.

Treatment of epilepsy by medication has been discussed at length earlier. It is worth repeating that for many people the taking of anti-epileptic medication is a protection against the recurrence of fits, in much the same way as some people have to take insulin to counteract adverse diabetic reactions. Once the type of medication and the satisfactory dose are arrived at, most people with epilepsy find that the medication makes very little difference to their everyday life and, as stated before, ideas of their being 'drug addicts' or 'under the influence of drugs' are inaccurate and unhelpful. Nevertheless, other people tend to ask embarrassing questions and give voice to all sorts of bizarre ideas about people who take drugs regularly.

Having to take tablets regularly may be an added problem to anyone seeking to take part in ordinary social activities. One young man reported that after a meal with a new girl friend he took out his pill box to take his mid-day dose. She expressed her astonishment, saying she thought it was only people who twitched who took pills. She seemed unconcerned about the epilepsy and thought he was quite normal because he did not twitch. Her mother might be much more concerned about the epilepsy and the prospect of her daughter having an 'epileptic' boy friend. Benny Jacobsen records that the mother of the first girl friend he wanted to marry upbraided him for thinking of marrying her daughter. She had thought him far too intelligent to suggest such a thing, and indeed she persuaded her daughter never to see him again.

Many states in the USA have had laws forbidding the marriage of people with epilepsy or requiring that they be sterilised if they wish to marry. Most of these laws have been repealed and where they do remain on the statute books they are no longer enforced. Similar laws were extant in Sweden until twenty years ago. Indeed, in the United Kingdom it was possible until 1970 for either party to obtain the annulment of a marriage within twelve months of the ceremony if the other had not disclosed a history of epilepsy. These laws were no doubt based on old ideas regarding the inheritance of epilepsy.

'Is it inherited?' is the question most frequently asked by any enquirer. The question is difficult to answer for the reason we have stressed earlier, that there is no single disease called epilepsy. Inheritance in some kinds of epilepsy may play a larger part than in others: for example, there is no evidence that a father who has developed epilepsy as a result of a head injury will have children subject to epilepsy: some mothers who had a tendency to convulsions in childhood may be more prone to have children with a tendency to convulsions or to minor epileptic attacks. One can only answer this question by quoting averages.

It seems that the risk of any child in the general population having epileptic attacks is about one in two hundred. Where one parent has epilepsy or has had epileptic attacks the risk appears to lie between three and ten in two hundred. Where both parents have epilepsy the risk may be much higher, but so much depends on the type of epilepsy, and at what age epileptic attacks began in each case, that figures are misleading. In all cases of doubt medical advice should be sought at a genetic advisory centre, to which reference can be made through the family doctor.

Having said all this, it must be admitted that adjustment to living with someone who is subject to epileptic attacks is not always easy. There may be need for good counselling from experienced people if the problems associated with epilepsy are not to assume too great an importance in the ordinary development of a successful marriage.

Another area in which old ideas of inheritance have still some influence is in the laws relating to immigration and citizenship of certain countries. A survey carried out several years ago revealed that many countries would not accept as prospective citizens people with a history of epileptic attacks. A more recent study shows many countries to have a much improved attitude, but there are still some sad exceptions. In Australia the Migration Act, Section 26, says that would-be immigrants must not have a 'proscribed disease', one of which is epilepsy. As a result of this policy the authorities imagine that there is no epilepsy in Australia. Unfortunately the facts belie this hope: Australia has its share of people with epilepsy, and local epilepsy associations exist to give help where needed. Detailed information about immigration prospects can be obtained from any of the epilepsy associations whose addresses are given in the Appendix.

One of the distressing aspects of being subject to epileptic attacks is the way in which one may be regarded as some sort of outcast. The Migration Act referred to above places epilepsy with scabies and any 'loathsome disease' among the proscribed diseases. An enquirer at South Africa House in London was once informed that everyone was welcomed in South Africa except 'hoboes, epileptics and drug addicts'. Fortunately such attitudes to epilepsy are now less common. A survey by Dr William Caveness of public attitudes towards epilepsy in the USA over twenty-five years showed that twenty-four per cent of people asked in 1949 would have objected to one of their children playing with a child who had seizures (fits). In 1974 only five per cent would have objected, and answers to other questions reflecting attitudes to the employment of people with epilepsy and the understanding of epilepsy have shown similar improvement over this period. There is, however, a constant need for programmes of public information and this is a major task of the epilepsy societies.

For too many years and for too many people a diagnosis of epilepsy has led to social isolation, either through direct rejection from membership of social groups or by voluntary withdrawal from such groups. In the first years of the activities of the British Epilepsy Association it was thought that epilepsy social clubs provided the alternative to such isolation but after a number of years these were often found to be too inward-looking. Some clubs continue to have an active and stimulating programme and provide much needed support, especially for the severely handicapped. In recent years the Association has developed an 'Action for Epilepsy' campaign and there are now more than a hundred local Action Groups throughout the country (including Northern Ireland). Interest in the development of such self-help groups has spread beyond the bounds of the United Kingdom. Certainly belonging to such groups where they meet other people with epilepsy or parents and families and understanding friends has made a great improvement in the lives of many people who formerly felt weighed down by all the complexities this diagnosis had meant for them. These groups have a dual role. They provide information for the local community in a great variety of ways and they offer support to individuals by sharing in the difficulties they may have to face.

In Britain, the position of people with epilepsy in the community has not been ignored by the appropriate government departments. Reference has already been made to the concern of the Department of Employment for the suitable employment of all disabled people. The health and welfare needs of people with epilepsy have been the subject of several studies. The last and most important has been the report of a special committee set up by the Department of Health and Social Security in 1967, published at the end of 1969. This report *People with Epilepsy*, can be considered a blue-print for the necessary services. Among its major recommendations were the following:

1. There should be a greater awareness that the possibilities for prevention, treatment and care in epilepsy have extended in recent years.
2. Further education about epilepsy should be directed to

health and social services personnel and also to the general public.

3. Epilepsy should no longer be a ground for the annulment of marriage.
4. Five or six special units for diagnosis and treatment, both medical and social, should be set up in England and Wales.
5. Unmarried mothers and people with epilepsy generally should not be debarred from residential social services.
6. Local authorities should provide hostel accommodation where necessary.
7. Services should be reviewed after five years.

The publication of this report was followed by national and regional conferences and there were great hopes that it would lead to a significant increase in the medical and social services for people with epilepsy, especially those with severe epilepsy. The establishment of more out-patient epilepsy clinics and the provision of more social services including hostel accommodation was confidently looked for. Unfortunately the economic recession of the early 1970s was not favourable to such expansion either in the hospital or social services and although many people still regard the report as an important milestone in the understanding of the needs of people with epilepsy they have had to accept more modest developments as a consequence of its appearance.

Three special centres have been recognised by the Department of Health. One which already existed in the hospital service in York, one which existed for children in Oxford, and a new experiment linking an old epilepsy colony at Chalfont with the National Hospital and Institute of Neurology at Queen Square in London. A review of the first five years has been carried out by the Department but the results are not yet available. Dr Maurice Parsonage, the Medical Director of the Centre in York, has written about the work at this centre (in the *Candle*, 1973) and pointed out that while there are many people with epilepsy of one kind or another who can manage to live happy and useful lives with just a little assistance, there is a small number of people whose need for special services arises from the complexity of their problems, where other handicaps make the treatment of epilepsy a great deal more difficult.

In many instances much work had to be done to define individual problems and these often involved families as well as patients. All the patients we admitted had long standing problems which had never before been properly defined, let alone solved. Virtually all our patients had employment problems of considerable magnitude. A recent assessment has shown that just about half of them were able to take up some kind of employment after discharge . . . Analysis of the reasons why employment problems could not be solved showed that handicaps other than epilepsy were the obstacles in all but two of the patients. In nearly two-thirds impairment of intellect provided the main source of difficulty, this usually being the result of brain damage sustained early on in life. Many times over, therefore, have we been reminded of the great need for the development of means of preventing this in future.

The Senior Physician at the Chalfont Centre introduced a description of those people needing the services of a special centre as those suffering from 'Epilepsy Plus'.

A fourth centre for epilepsy is developing outside the experiment supported by the Department of Health. A one-time epilepsy colony in Cheshire has secured support from the Regional Authority to develop a more forward-looking therapeutic epilepsy centre. We are still some way short of the proposals of the *People with Epilepsy* report. It is hoped that the impetus gained from its publication will not be lost altogether because many people who have to live with epilepsy and whose problems are not so complex as defined above would gain a great deal if there were a better understanding of epilepsy and its accompanying difficulties.

CHAPTER 10

Some Further Advice

Before concluding this 'plain man's guide to epilepsy' we thought we should ask some people with epilepsy what they felt about living with this condition. Sometimes there is a great deal of similarity in their comments but sometimes there is a wide divergence emphasising once again that a 'typical epileptic' does not exist.

Penny is a highly intelligent, charming and determined young lady who has had epileptic fits for the past ten years. In spite of a number of obstacles - one of which is the regrettable tendency to have fits now and again - she has got herself through college to follow the course she set her heart on. When asked what she thought teachers should be told about people with epilepsy she replied: 'Don't let the child get away with it.' There was no question of her feeling deprived or frustrated if she was not taken to the swimming baths with the rest of the class. She disliked the baths and disliked swimming and used her epilepsy to escape an unpleasant activity. She thinks that her teachers were too readily persuaded to let her 'get away with it' on this and other occasions.

Penny feels that teachers and all adults should be more honest and truthful. One of her more painful memories was of being denied the chance of an exchange visit to a French family when she was twelve. She was told: 'It is a pity that we cannot find someone with whom you can exchange.' What hurt her most was the discovery that the teachers were not prepared to advance her application, but asked her mother to fob her off with a half-truth. Penny, being the determined person she is, eventually obtained an exchange through another channel.

How does one tell people one has epilepsy, and when does one tell them? Does one walk into a room and say, 'Hullo everyone, I'm Penny, I have fits.' Should one wear a badge or a patch on one's coat so that everyone knows that there is 'something different about me'? She admits that there is no easy answer, and of course she is not alone in this. Because she has three or four fits a year and sometimes more in new circumstances, Penny makes a point of telling an adult at work or at college that she is liable to attacks. She does this mainly because she does not want to be taken off to hospital and is proud of the fact that she has not yet seen the inside of an ambulance – at least not as a patient.

Her boy friend knows about her attacks. On one occasion she had a fit in the street when she was out with him. She came round to hear him doing his best to reassure passers-by that an ambulance was not required. Penny usually becomes aware of her surroundings very soon after the seizure is over, but for as long as ten or fifteen minutes she may be able to see or hear what is going on without being able to speak clearly. In this state she once heard someone ask: 'What has she been drinking?' This made her very angry and the memory still rankles.

In our experience people who conceal, or attempt to conceal, their fits are often criticised. It is plainly ill-advised to deny the existence of fits which occur frequently and without warning. On the other hand, it is highly debatable whether we should expect someone who has not had any form of attack for five years or more to place himself at a disadvantage when applying for employment by declaring that he has epilepsy. There can be no hard and fast rule, but it seems that a reasonable reticence should be acceptable.

Further advice from Penny related to what to do when faced with someone having an epileptic fit. Her first words were: 'Don't panic'. Most fits are short-lived and unless she is in real danger of harming herself she prefers to be left to 'do my own thing'. Almost everyone who has epilepsy has little idea what a major seizure looks like. Penny is no exception and she was puzzled why people made so much fuss or why they were so upset. It is perhaps necessary to point out to people with epilepsy that the major seizure is distressing and frightening to the observer. Perhaps because modern treatment has reduced the number of fits which occur, fewer people have seen a fit and more people imagine the underlying sequence of events to be far more serious than it really is.

In this respect Penny remembers with particular gratitude the girl who, after seeing Penny have an attack at college, said she did not know why there was so much fuss about epileptic fits. In contrast to this attitude she complains that some people go out of their way to be over-attentive and over-careful on her behalf. This she finds a great deal more embarrassing than coping with people who don't want to have anything to do with her or her epilepsy.

Certain words rankle. 'I do not *suffer* from epilepsy,' said Julie one evening. Julie had quite a lot of trouble with epileptic attacks before she achieved control of them. She has also had domestic upheavals in her life. She has a regular and important job and is always prepared to help when voluntary help is wanted. She dislikes being thought of as a 'sufferer' from epilepsy – as well she might.

Some people dislike the word 'fit'. They feel this is degrading or in some way frightening. They prefer black-outs, turns or attacks.

There are mixed feelings about calling oneself 'an epileptic'. Doctors and social workers usually avoid speaking of someone as 'an epileptic' since such a label is difficult to define accurately – we are all more or less epileptic – and it is also socially harmful. And yet some people seem to have no hesitation in saying 'I am an epileptic'. A short time ago a young man asked one of us to tell him what was the definition of an epileptic. He resented being told he was one. He was thirty-five years of age. He had had epileptic fits between the ages of four years and ten years. Following brain surgery he had not had an attack for twenty-five years. Was he an epileptic?

In 1977 the International Epilepsy Congress in Holland devoted an afternoon to listening to a group of people talking about what epilepsy had meant in their lives. The group consisted of a married couple (the husband has epilepsy), a young man and a young woman and two sets of parents each of whom had a child with epilepsy. A full report can be obtained from the British Epilepsy Association. Some of the thoughts expressed were:

'Passing examinations and other successes in life in spite of having epilepsy gives one a greater sense of achievement.'

'When the doctor said "he has got epilepsy" I felt as if my world had come to an end because I knew nothing about it.'

'I tried to shut it out of my mind. It was only when I obtained a place in a British team that I had to face up to it and ever since I have been very glad that I have faced up to it.'

'One father said the uncertainty was the worst part of epilepsy. Would his boy be all right when riding his bicycle or swimming or just going to the local shop?'

'One can never really relax.'

'Children adapt quickly to father having an attack.'

'Children at school very soon take it for granted once they know one has epileptic attacks.'

'Stress in athletics and in training makes little difference but one always feels the need to take extra care about getting the right amount of sleep and not eating or drinking too much.'

'Being married to someone with epilepsy is just like being married to anybody else.'

'I sometimes feel that I am slowed up by my drugs.'

'I don't think it [anti-epileptic medication] makes any difference to me, but often I would like to find out by putting myself off drugs and seeing whether I would come out a different me at the other end.'

'Yes, I'd really like to know what I was really like without the tablets.'

'As far as epilepsy and society is concerned, I have thought a lot about this and I feel myself very definitely a second-class citizen in the eyes of society.'

So what does all this mean? What have we been trying to say in this introduction to epilepsy?

Professor Pond once said that to be any real help to someone who has a complex epileptic disorder one really had to be 'hooked on epilepsy'. Not all cases of epilepsy are complex and not everyone wants to be deeply involved in epilepsy. We do not insist that everyone should become a specialist in epilepsy in regard to either the medical or social aspects. We do ask that people should realise that epilepsy is of general concern. As soon as one looks around in an understanding and helpful way one finds that epilepsy affects more people's lives than one had expected. Recently, after lecturing to students one morning, the writer called at a local shop for a small purchase and discovered that the shop keeper had a seventeen-year-old son with epilepsy who had left school and needed help in finding an occupation, and that the shop assistant's mother had a mild form of epilepsy. Experiences like this are not rare if one is ready to listen and become aware of some of the problems.

Penny makes light of her epilepsy, but for many others it is catastrophic to have seizures. To have an experience which others do not seem to understand makes one feel very much alone. The opportunity to talk over the difficulties quietly and without fuss is of tremendous importance to many patients and parents. We hope that this book will persuade social workers to seek out study days organised by local epilepsy associations and other means of being better informed for such counselling, as well as putting their clients in touch with their local group.

We hope also that teachers will not only see the importance of knowing something more about epilepsy, but will appreciate the value of treating the child with epileptic attacks quietly and calmly. In this way, not only does the child himself learn to come to terms with his disability, but the other children may grow up prepared to accept epilepsy as a part of life.

Parents often feel that they are told more than they can remember or that the questions they wish to ask are never answered. We hope that some of the answers are in this book. If not, seek out your epilepsy association and local Action Group for informative literature: raise questions with your social worker, who may have more time than the physician to answer them. Do make sure that the simple rules of treatment are fully understood: when to take tablets and the importance of making changes only when medical advice has been obtained.

People who have epilepsy have a duty to themselves to obtain the best possible advice. If your general practitioner prescribes medication and your seizures become controlled there does not appear to be any need for further advice on this score. If you obtain congenial employment and you experience no social difficulties it is clearly best to get on with leading a normal life and be satisfied with good results. If things do not go so well it may be necessary to ask the general practitioner to refer you to a medical specialist. If there are difficulties in finding work, the advice of the DRO should be sought, or a social services department should be consulted if other social problems arise. Do not accept problems until you are quite sure nothing further can be done. Make sure you have followed up all the possibilities which exist to help the disabled person both at work and at home. If you are in any doubt consult your Epilepsy Association.

Above all, it is important that someone with epilepsy should not believe that every single thing that goes amiss in his daily life is due to the epileptic attacks. Someone with no aptitude for book-keeping or for carpentry or for an academic career should not be encouraged to follow a wrongly chosen occupation and then blame his difficulties on epilepsy. We are all subject to disappointments in life whether we have epilepsy or not, and we can all be dissatisfied with the job, disenchanted by the employer or uninspired by the teacher. Earlier in this book we urged employers to see epilepsy in proper perspective when thinking of a possible employee. It is equally important that people with epilepsy see their disability in proper perspective and do not let it run their lives. Furthermore, understanding the difficulties of the other person is a two-way process. There are times when it is just as necessary for someone with a disability to make allowances for the non-disabled. Some people are embarrassed by disability and find it difficult to behave in a normal way towards the disabled person.

Epilepsy has been known through the ages. The myths and misunderstandings which it has collected are not likely to disappear from men's minds after one publicity drive. Nor will the acceptance of epilepsy be achieved by any one-sided approach. Scientific research into epilepsy has to be multi-faceted and multi-disciplinary. Social acceptance needs the concerted action of people with epilepsy as well as those of us who have not yet experienced our first epileptic attack. There are signs that public attitudes towards epilepsy have improved in recent years and many people with epilepsy are determined that they will not let epilepsy interfere with their lives. It is our hope that joint action will finally lay the bogey of the falling sickness.

Suggestions for Further Reading

Bower Brian and Ward, Francesca. *A Study of Certain Social Aspects of Epilepsy in Childhood.* Published by Spastic International Medical Publications, London 1978.

Epilepsy in Society. London: Office of Health Economics, 1971.

Livingstone, Samuel. *Living with Epileptic Seizures.* Springfield, Ill.: Charles C. Thomas, 1963.

A New Look at Life by People with Epilepsy. Published by Epilepsy International, Washington 1978. Obtainable from the British Epilepsy Association, Wokingham, Berks.

People with Epilepsy. Report from the Department of Health and Social Security. London: HMSO, 1969.

Pond, Desmond and Johnson, Eric. *Epilepsy and Fits.* Family Doctor Booklet. London: British Medical Association, 1965, revised, 1973.

Pryse-Phillips, William. *Epilepsy.* Bristol, John Wright, 1969.

Scott, Donald. *About Epilepsy,* London: Duckworth 1969, revised, 1973 & 1978.

Sutherland, J. M. and Tait, H. *The Epilepsies: Modern Diagnosis and Treatment.* Edinburgh: Livingstone, 1969, revised, 1974, with the assistance of Eadie, H. J.

Appendix: Some Useful Addresses

Information about national and local associations in most parts of the world is available from:

>The International Bureau for Epilepsy
>c/o The David Lewis Centre
>Alderley Edge
>Cheshire SK9 7UD
>England

The leading national associations of the English-speaking countries are given below:

AUSTRALIA

Epileptic Welfare Association
of Queensland
Room 511, Fifth Floor
Pennys Building
210 Queen Street
Brisbane
Queensland 4000

Epileptic Welfare Association
PO Box 221
North Sydney
NSW 2060

Epilepsy Social Welfare Foundation
Clark Rubber Building, Third Floor
196 Flinders Street
Melbourne
Victoria 3000

AUSTRALIA (cont.)   Epilepsy Association of
South Australia, Inc.
PO Box 252
Glenelg
SA 5045

West Australian Epilepsy Association
14 Bagot Road
Subiaco
WA 6008

CANADA   Edmonton Epilepsy Association
725 Tegler Building
Edmonton 15
Alberta

Epilepsy Association of Calgary
2422 5th Avenue NW
Calgary
Alberta T2N 0T2

British Columbia Epilepsy
Association
1195 West 8th Avenue
Vancouver
BC V6H 1C5

Epilepsy Canada and
Ontario Epilepsy Association
90 Eglinton Avenue East
Suite 405
Toronto
Ontario

Epilepsy Association Metro-Toronto
Suite 510
1260 Bay Street
Toronto
Ontario M5R 2B1

GREAT BRITAIN	British Epilepsy Association Crowthorne House Bigshotte New Wokingham Road Wokingham Berks RG1 3AY
	Northern Ireland Region (of British Epilepsy Association) Claremont Street Hospital Claremont Street Belfast BT9 6AQ
	Scottish Epilepsy Association 48 Govan Road Glasgow GS1 1JL
	Epilepsy Association of Edinburgh and SE Region 13 Guthrie Street Edinburgh EH1 1JG
INDIA	Indian Epilepsy Association 251 D.Naoroji Road Bombay 400001
IRISH REPUBLIC	Irish Epilepsy Association 23 Dawson Street Dublin 2 Republic of Ireland
NEW ZEALAND	New Zealand Epilepsy Association PO Box 683 Hamilton
SOUTH AFRICA	South African National Epilepsy League PO Box 4197 Pretoria 0001

USA   Epilepsy Foundation of America
           Suite 406
           1828 L. Street NW
           Washington DC 20036

Index